D0605023

NURSE

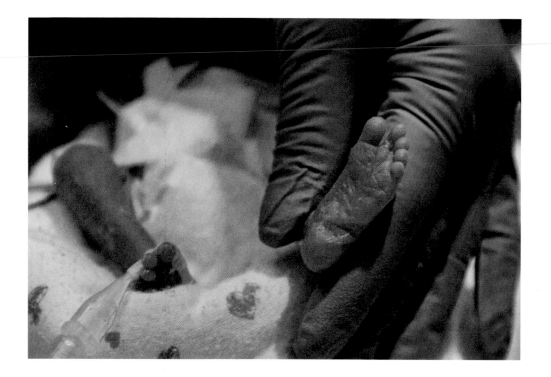

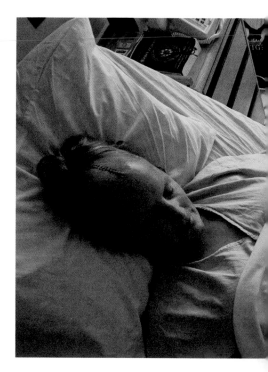

TO NURTURE

TO CARE

BY PETER JARET   SENIOR EDITOR MARLA SALMON

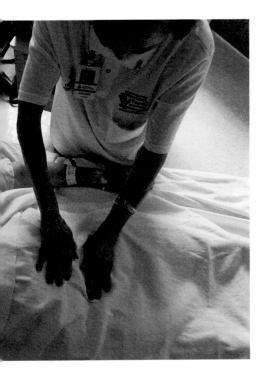
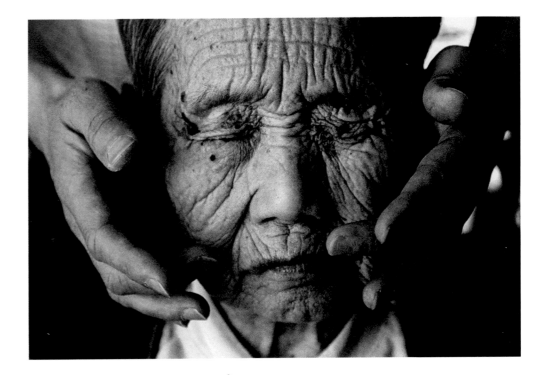

TO BE A NURSE

PHOTOGRAPHS BY KAREN KASMAUSKI

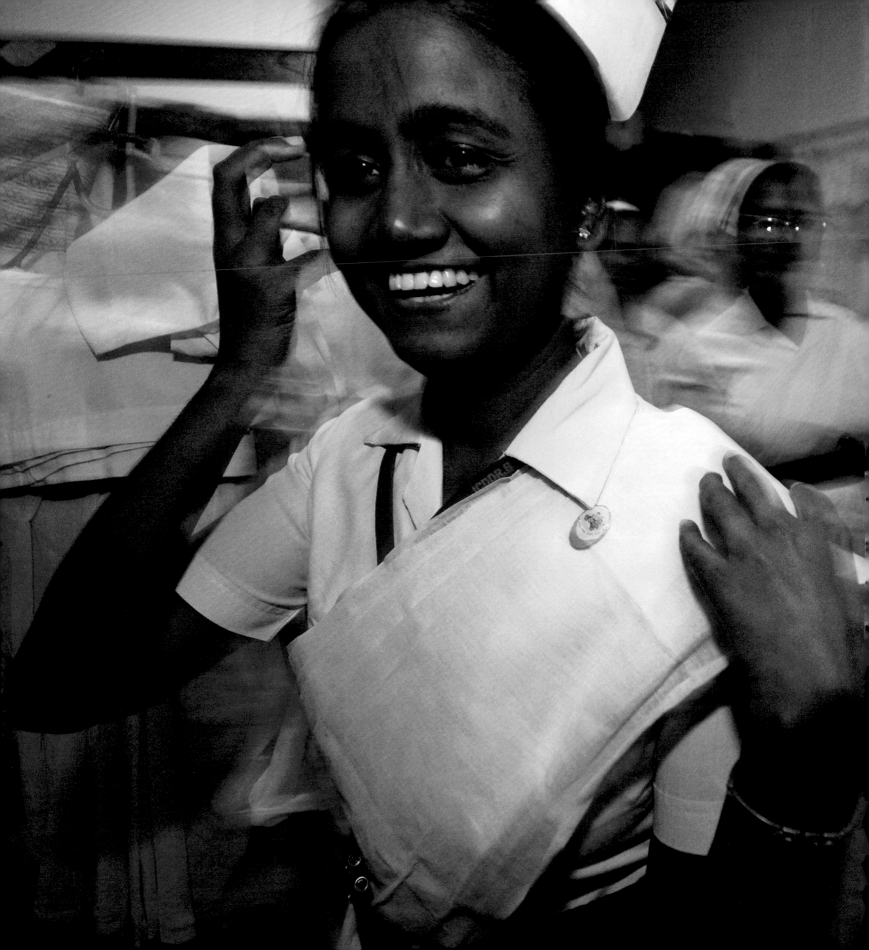

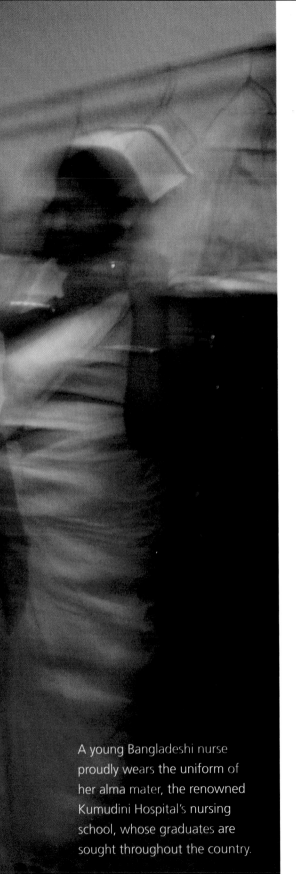

A young Bangladeshi nurse proudly wears the uniform of her alma mater, the renowned Kumudini Hospital's nursing school, whose graduates are sought throughout the country.

CONTENTS

THE POWER TO MAKE A DIFFERENCE

BY JIMMY CARTER

I grew up with nurses. My mother, Lillian Carter, was a nurse, and as a boy I was often in the company of the nurses she worked with in Plains, Georgia. I saw how incredibly hard they labored—12-hour days for the princely sum of four dollars, as I recall—and I witnessed firsthand the enormous contribution they made to our small community.

I did not understand then, of course, how much nursing would inspire me in my own life. In a time of racial segregation, my mother treated everyone alike and spent many hours nursing our black neighbors. Later, at the age of 68, she joined the Peace Corps and for almost two years worked in India, where she cared for many seriously ill people, including patients with leprosy. It was, I know, one of the most meaningful experiences of her life.

Throughout her life, Lillian Carter was a woman of strong ideals and almost limitless energy. She was, in short, a nurse—someone who believed deeply that the highest manifestation of her faith was to care for those in need. The work of nursing is to alleviate unnecessary suffering and pain, to give people not only health and hope but also self-respect. Underlying that mission is the belief that everyone deserves a fair chance at a healthy life. Freedom from unnecessary disease and suffering is not something for the privileged few, after all. It is a basic human right.

Tragically, it is a right that far too few people around the world enjoy.

That is why it is so important for all of us to support nurses and the courageous work they do. Health is only part of it. Guided by the belief that everyone deserves care and compassion, nurses fight against discrimination and stigmatization. They reach across the widening chasm between rich and poor. They break down the other walls that too often separate people—religion, nationality, race, and gender—to affirm the essence of humanity

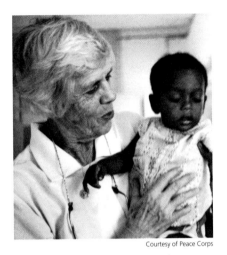

Lillian Carter in India during her Peace Corps days.

that joins all of us. They crusade for healthy communities and wider access to basic health care for everyone. They understand the incredible power one person can have to make a difference in the lives of others. The very best of them, like my mother, inspire others to carry on the great work of nursing.

My mother certainly inspired me. At The Carter Center, we work on many fronts to improve the health of individuals and communities, to nourish hope and self-respect. Our programs target neglected diseases in some of the world's most impoverished and forgotten communities. In six nations in sub-Saharan African we are battling trachoma, the leading cause of preventable blindness in the world. In Nigeria we are working to spare people the debilitating fevers and disfigurement of lymphatic filariasis, spread by mosquitoes. In Ethiopia we launched the Public Health Training Initiative that, in partnership with seven Ethiopian universities, developed new health curricula to train health officials, workers, and teachers. Our efforts depend on a strong and committed network of nurses and health care workers. Their dedication continues to inspire us, each and every day, to achieve the highest moral value embodied by nursing: reaching out to those most in need.

Our partner in this work, the Lillian Carter Center for International Nursing in the school of nursing at Emory University, has been instrumental in bringing nursing's global contributions and challenges to the forefront. Hence, the significance of this book. It is about the kind of work nurses around the world do every day—that my mother did in our small community in Georgia and in a village in India. It serves to remind us that nurses embody what is most precious in humankind. When the world at large comes to value the contributions of nurses, it also will embrace its most vulnerable people, those whom nurses seek to serve.

THE VOICE OF NURSING

BY MARLA SALMON

This book is deeply personal for me. It is rooted in a need that has haunted me for three decades as a nurse—to shine a light on what too often remains invisible: the crucial work of nurses around the world. To give voice to those who usually reserve their own voices for speaking out on behalf of others.

My work has traversed the landscape of caring, from touching those who are suffering to teaching those who will become nurses. I have collaborated with nurses around the world in order to shape national and global health policy, and I've seen firsthand the many ways that nursing promotes health and hope, often under difficult and even dangerous circumstances. I've also seen it in my personal life. My mother was a nurse. My daughter is a nurse. Yet, despite all I've learned as a nurse, working on this book moved me in ways I didn't expect. What began as an attempt to document nursing's contribution around the world ended up as something much more: a sweeping tapestry of humanity itself.

There are the unforgettable images. Of the tenderness in the face of a nurse-brother in Jamaica bathing an emaciated young man with AIDS. Of the camaraderie and excitement of young nursing students helping one another with their uniforms, the identity of their new profession. Of a community joining together to embrace those whom illness has stigmatized, captured in the images of a coffee ceremony in Ethiopia.

And the voices. Of the public health nurse in Cuba who goes door to door, returning again and again until she has reached everyone in a rural community. Of the school nurse in Arizona who devotes her days off providing emergency care to immigrants crossing dangerous stretches of desert in search of better prospects. Of the nurses in Kenya who

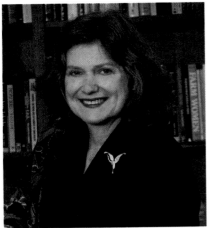
Steve Ellwood

volunteer their time to care for people with AIDS in the poorest slums.

Together, they create a vivid portrait of who we are at our best. Nursing, after all, is motivated by the finest impulse of humanity—to care for others, even those different from ourselves. In modern nursing, that impulse is given strength and sinew by professional training and the expertise that comes from a growing body of nursing research.

This book, then, is a tribute to nurses. And an urgent plea. Today, at a time when nursing offers a solution to so many of the world's most pressing health care challenges, the profession that is synonymous with caring is itself in need of care. Nursing shortages, difficult and dangerous working conditions, lack of respect and autonomy—all threaten the work of nurses. In many places, the fragile bond of caring that ties us together—the bond that expresses itself in nursing—is in real danger.

That should concern us all. Nursing is a societal good. There will come a time when practically every one of us will depend on the care of a nurse. It's up to each of us to take note of this precious resource and ensure that nursing receives the resources and respect it needs.

I hope this book will serve to inspire and inform reflection and action—and help guarantee that when a nurse is needed, he or she will be there to serve, care, innovate, advocate, discover, comfort, nurture, educate, and partner in the fundamental human process of caring.

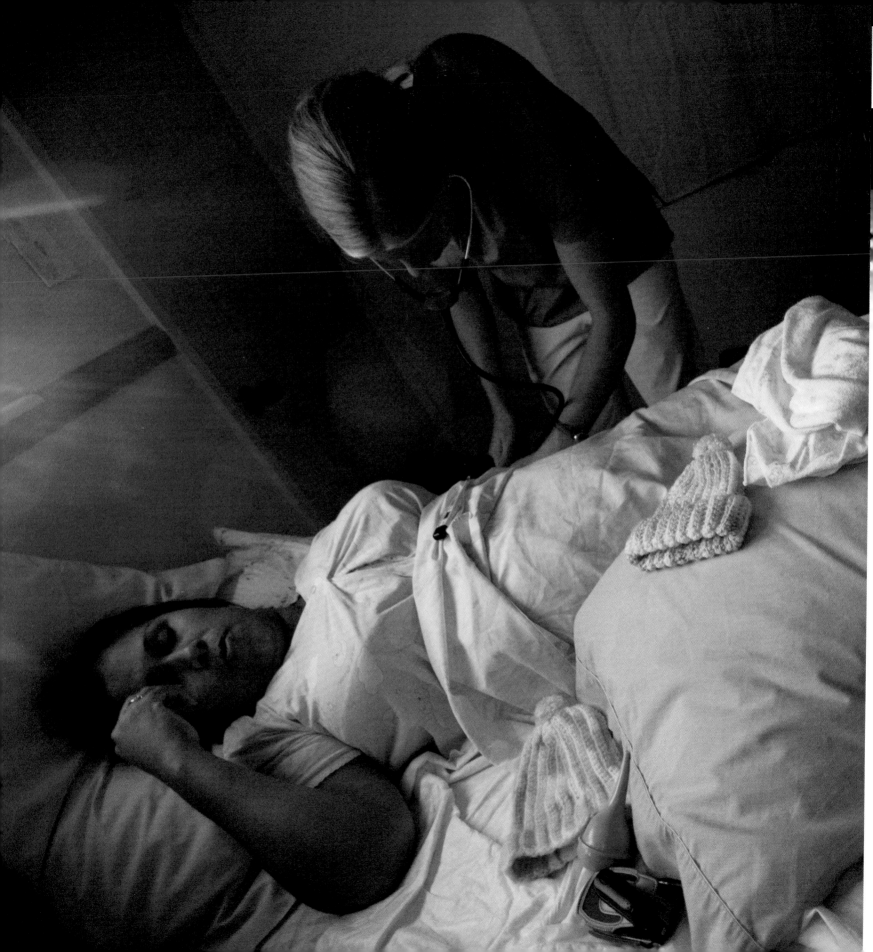

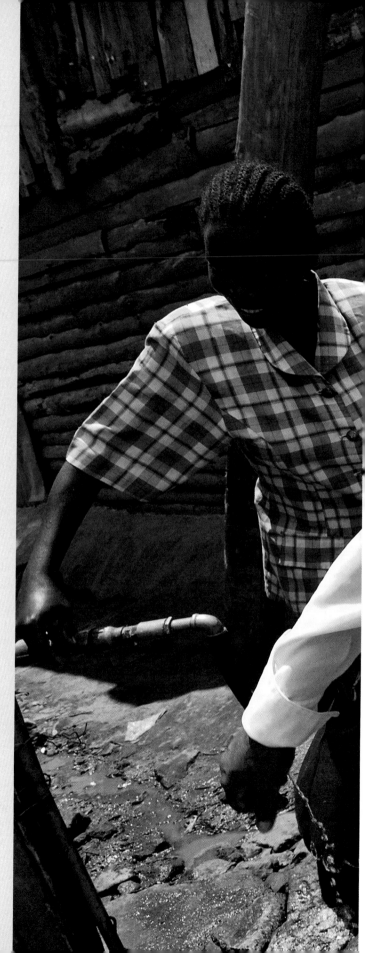

PASSAGES OF LIFE

A PORTFOLIO

In one of the sprawling slums of Nairobi, Kenya, a retired hospital nurse now volunteers as a community outreach nurse, helping AIDS patients and their families cope with the disease.

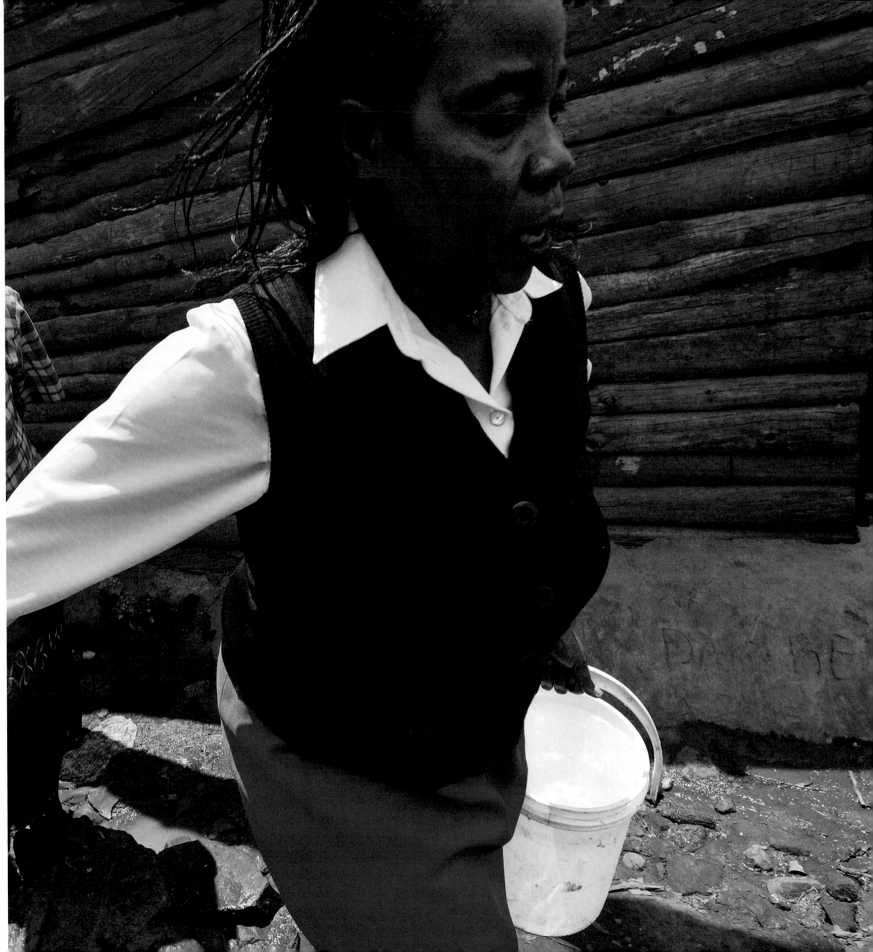

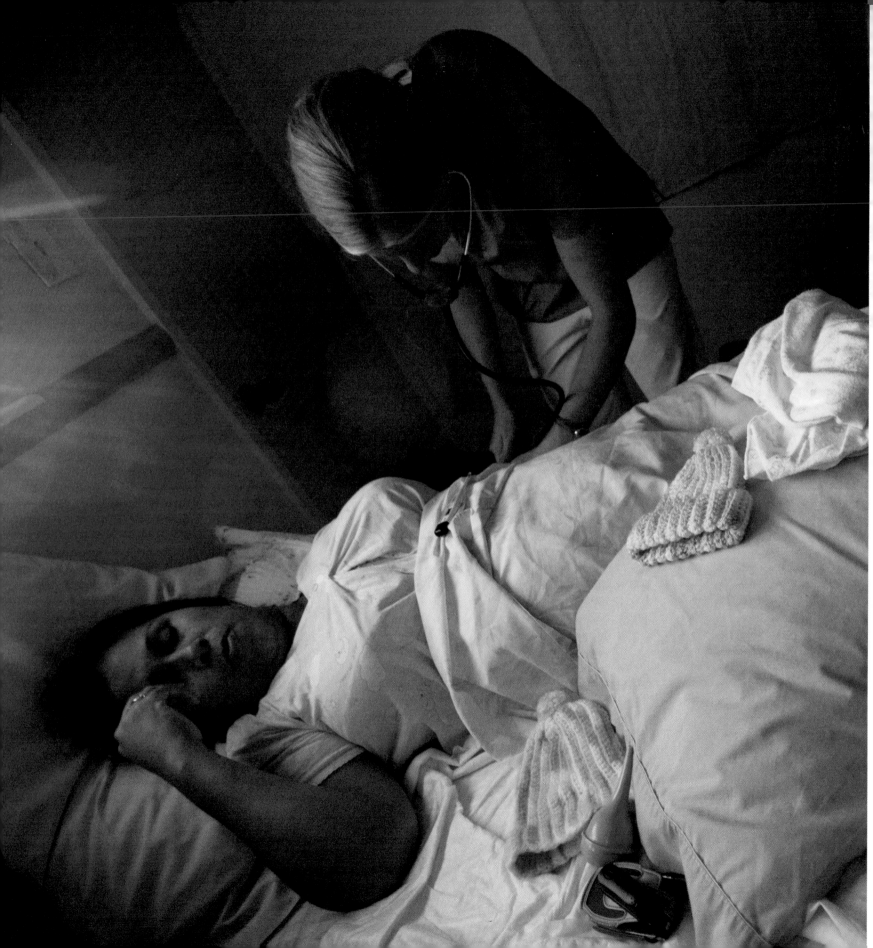

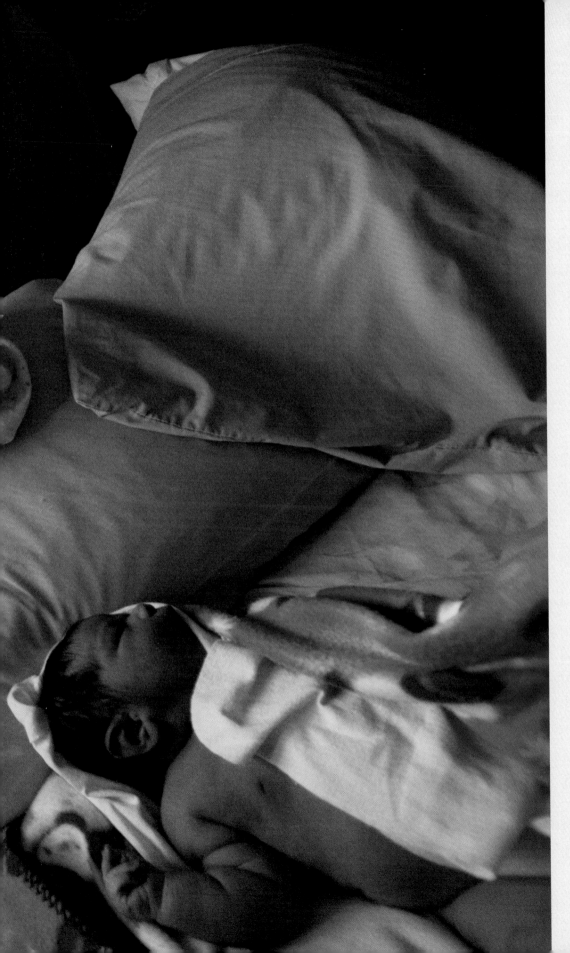

A mother and her newborn rest comfortably, thanks to the competent care of a nurse midwife at the Holy Family Birth Center in Weslaco, Texas. An ancient and respected art, midwifery is a well-recognized nursing practice in many parts of the world.

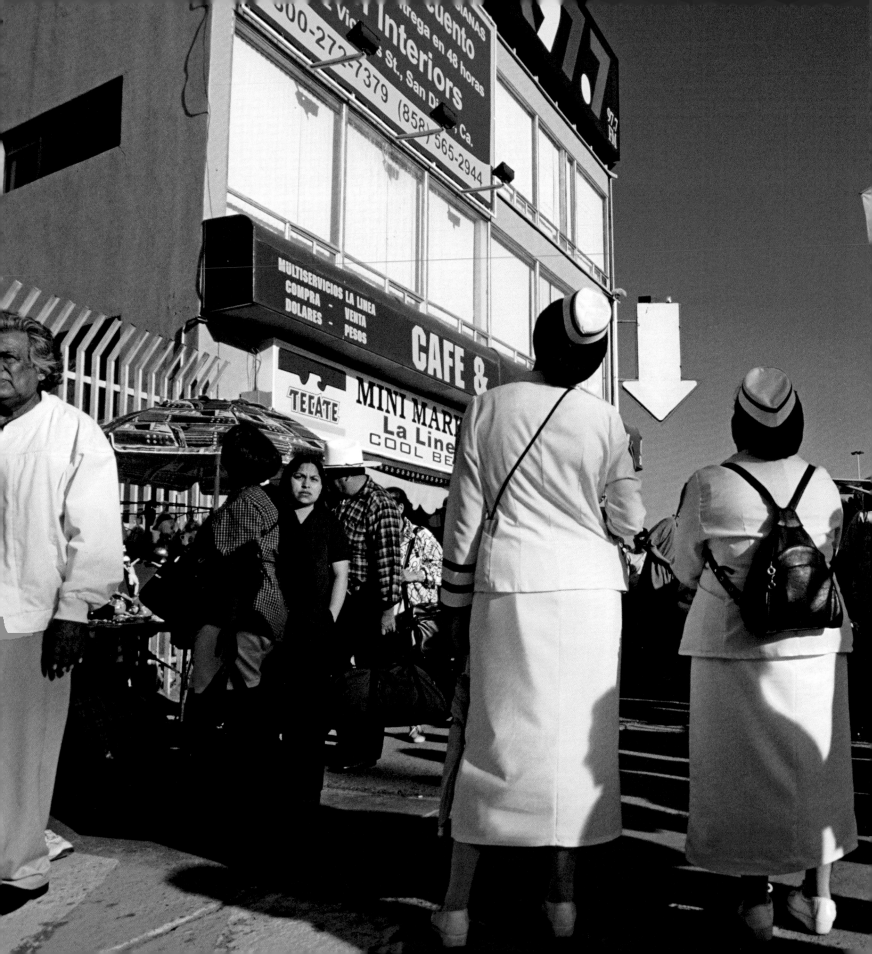

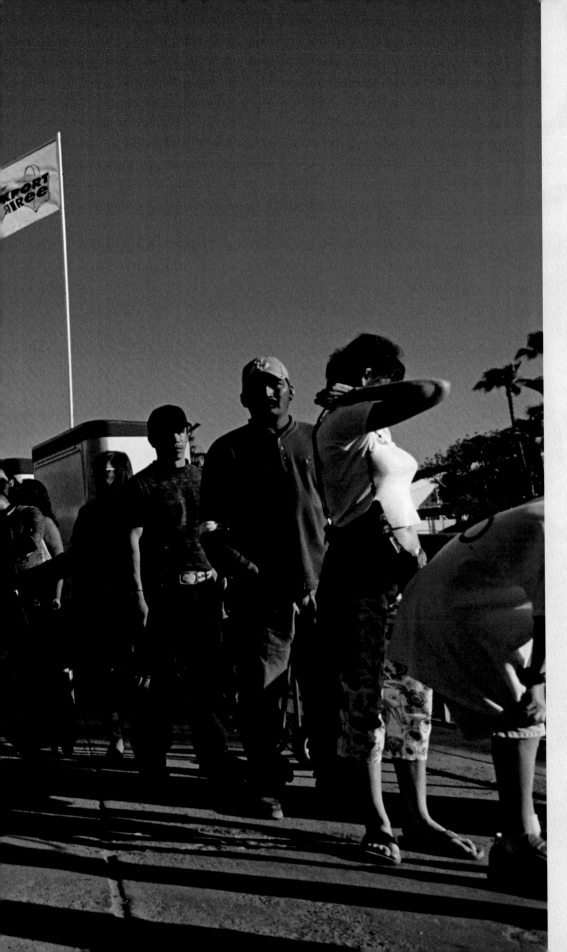

Mexican nurses mingle with the crowds in Tijuana, one of the many border towns worldwide where health issues require cooperation across country boundaries. Just as diseases—in this city, particularly tuberculosis—know no boundaries, neither does the commitment of nurses to provide care, regardless of nationality or geopolitics.

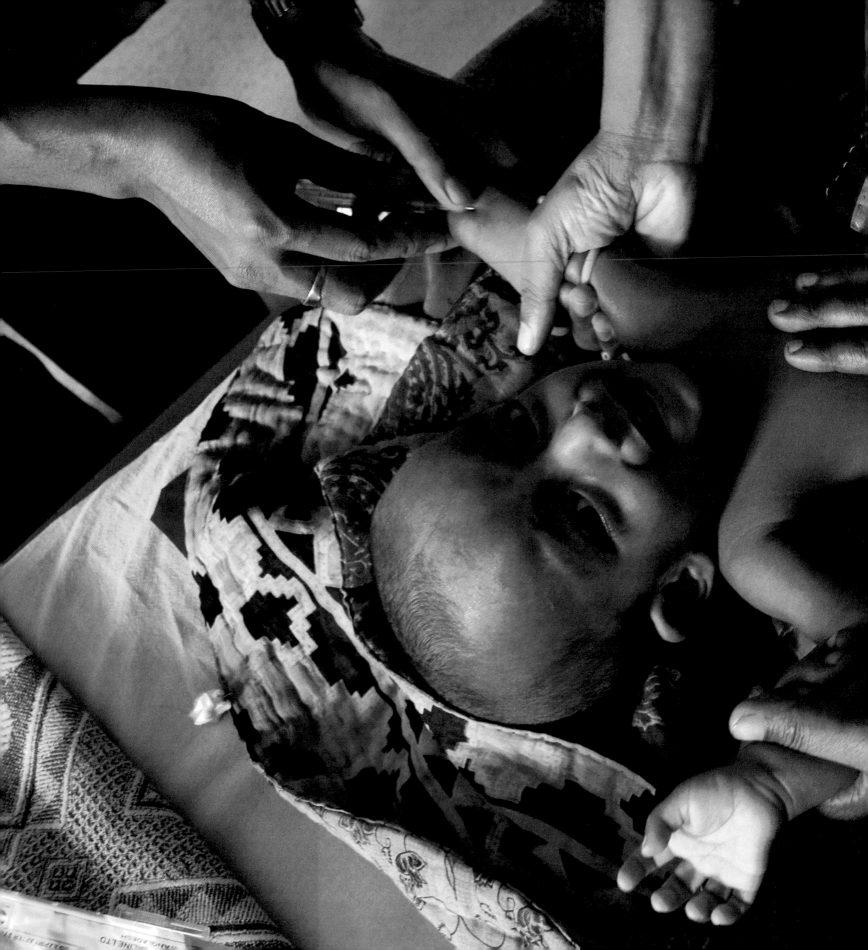

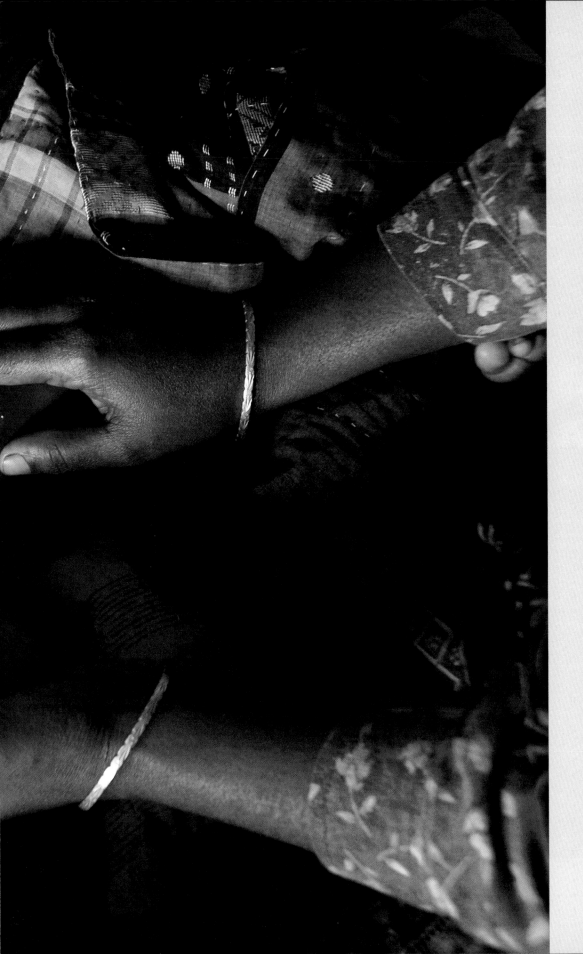

At Kumudini Hospital in Narayanganj, Bangladesh, a nursing student inoculates a young child as her preceptor looks on. Inexpensive vaccines, so critical to childhood health, require the presence of nurses to administer them—and in many poorer countries, that presence is too often lacking.

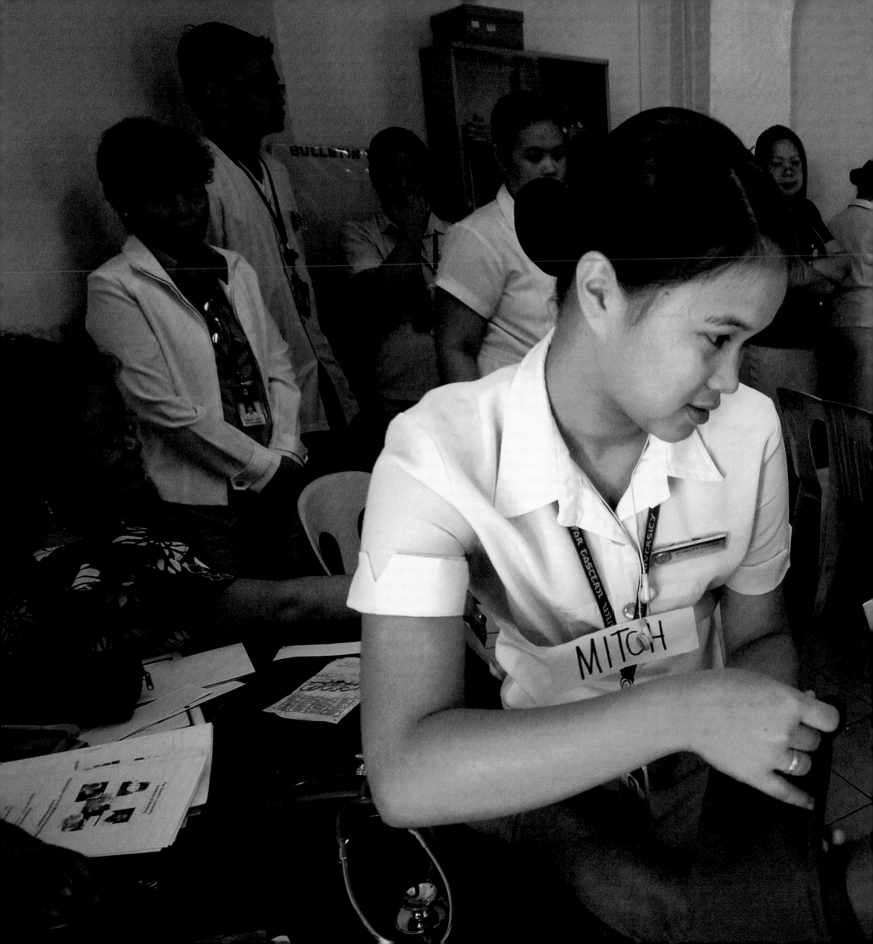

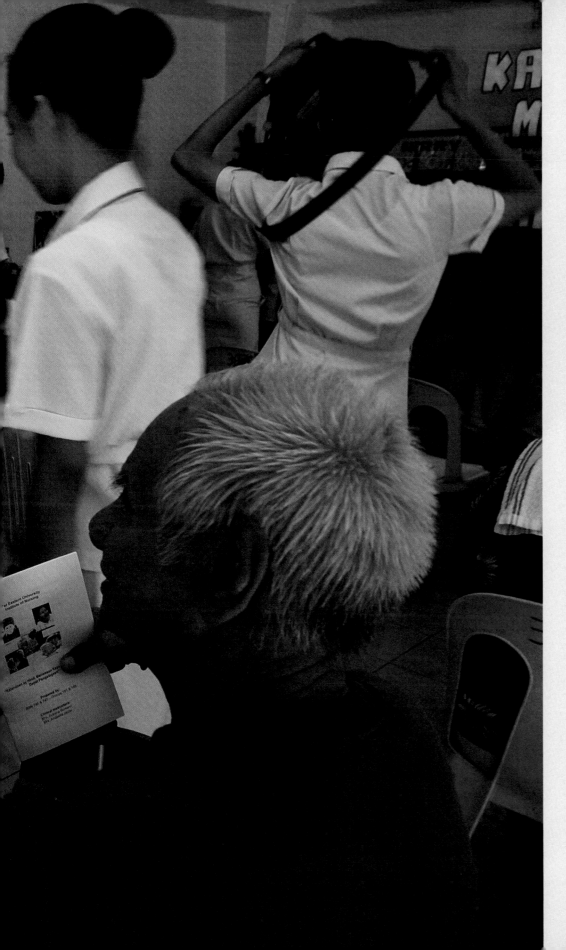

A scene found around the world—young nurses caring for the elderly. This Filipina nursing student is taking a man's blood pressure in Manila, and just as important, giving him her full attention. As much as technical know-how, nursing is about nurturing and listening.

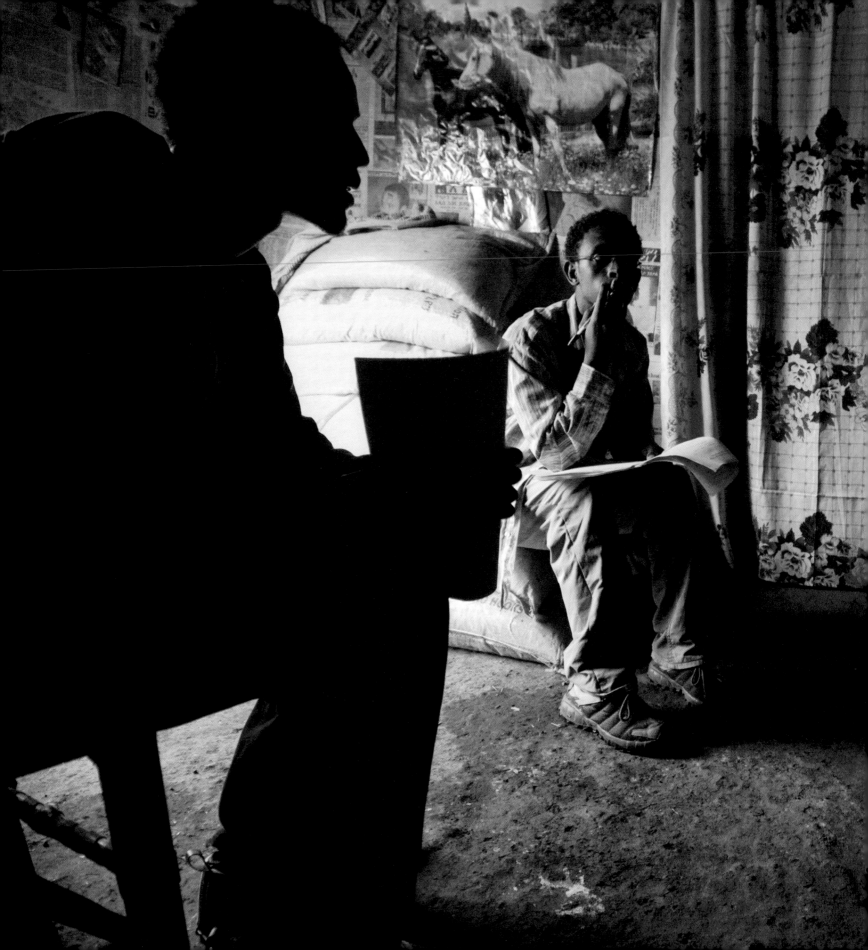

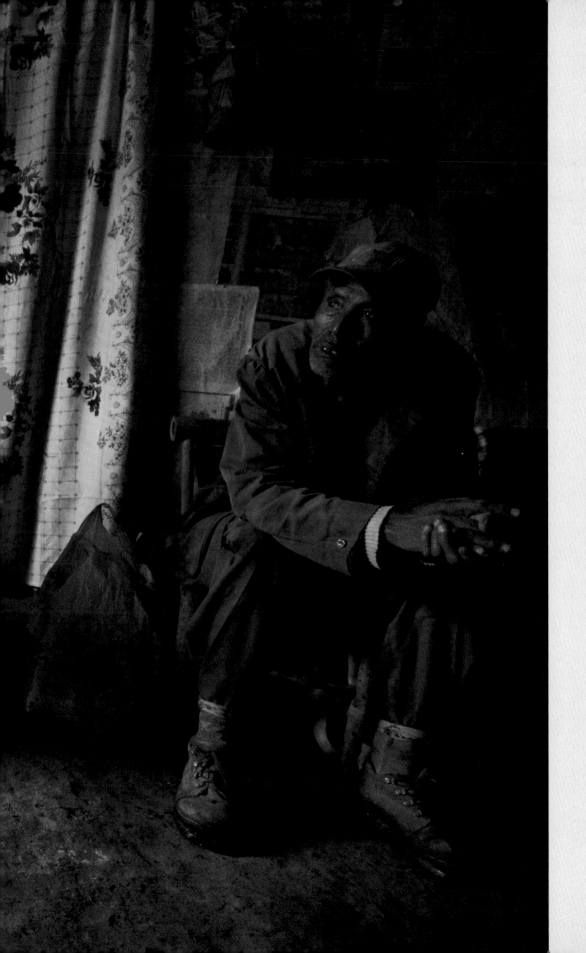

Taking a health survey, nursing students in Sendafa, Ethiopia, interview a resident (on the right) in his simple home, where he lives without benefit of running water or electricity. In some African cultures, male nurses, relatively well paid and well respected, are common.

Village health care volunteers like Shahnaz have changed the face of medicine in rural Bangladesh. Trained in basic nursing skills and supervised by a health care professional, Shahnaz treats her fellow villagers, who would otherwise have little opportunity for care.

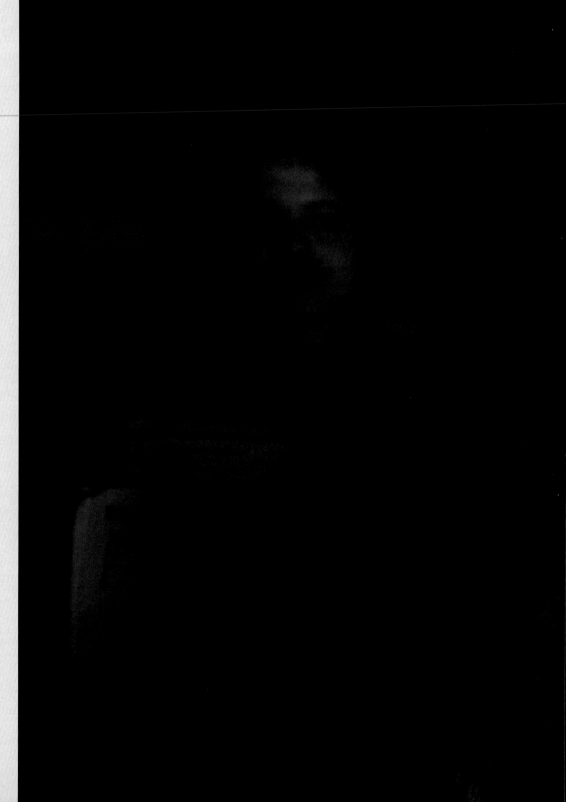

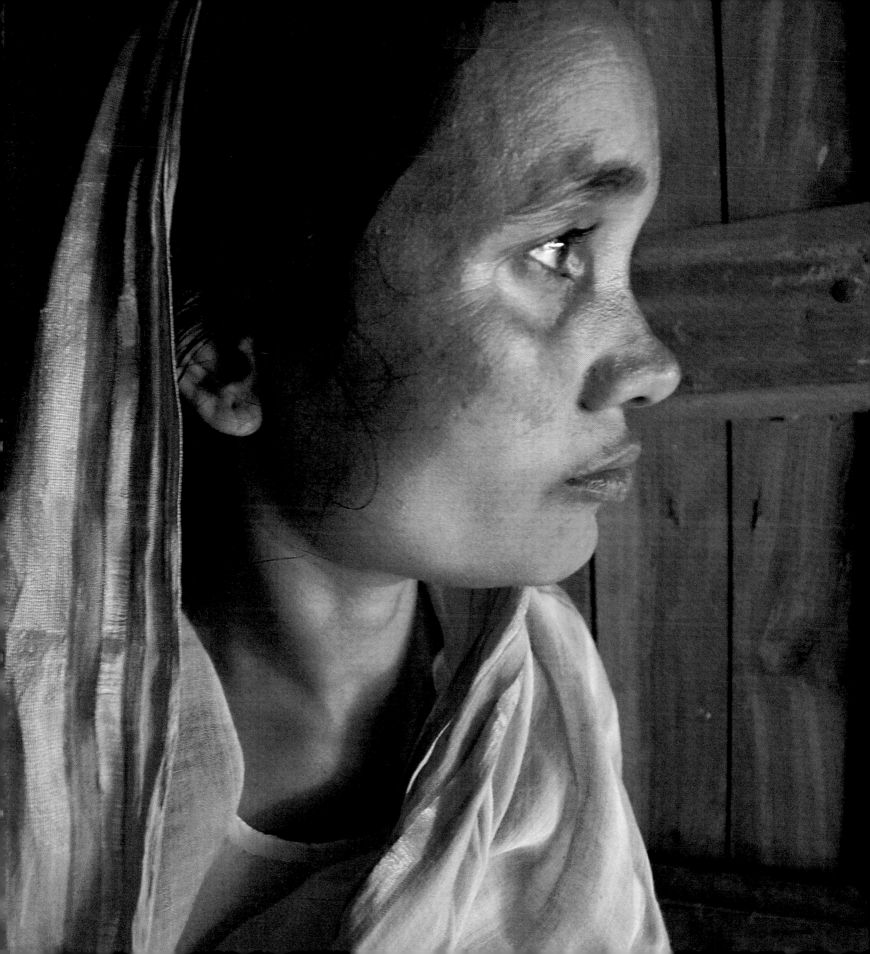

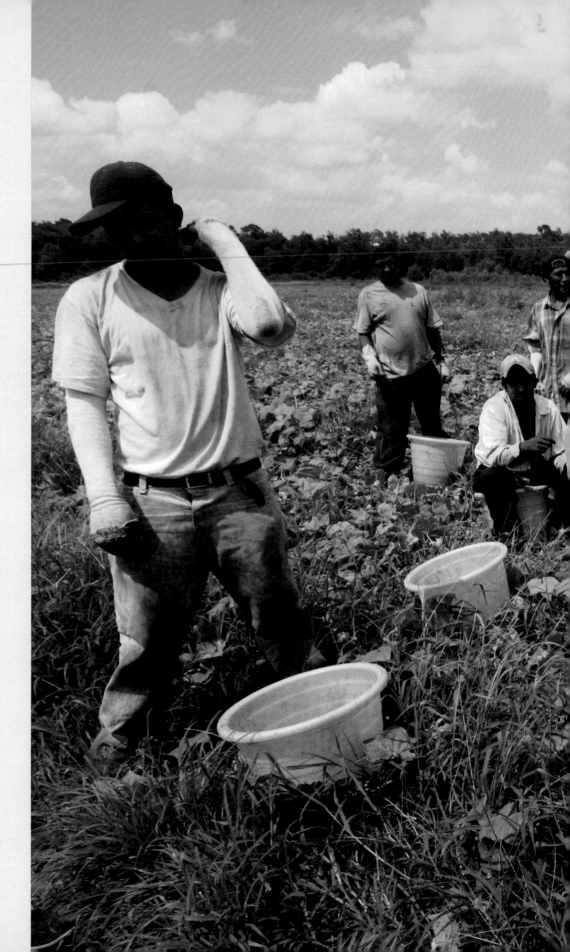

Nurses go where the need is, and every June students and faculty at Emory University's Nell Hodgson Woodruff School of Nursing in Atlanta take their skills into the farm fields of Georgia to offer check-ups and other care to more than a thousand migrant workers and their families. For many of them, this is the only health care they'll receive the entire year. Wordwide, medical attention for the growing numbers of migrating people has become a real challenge.

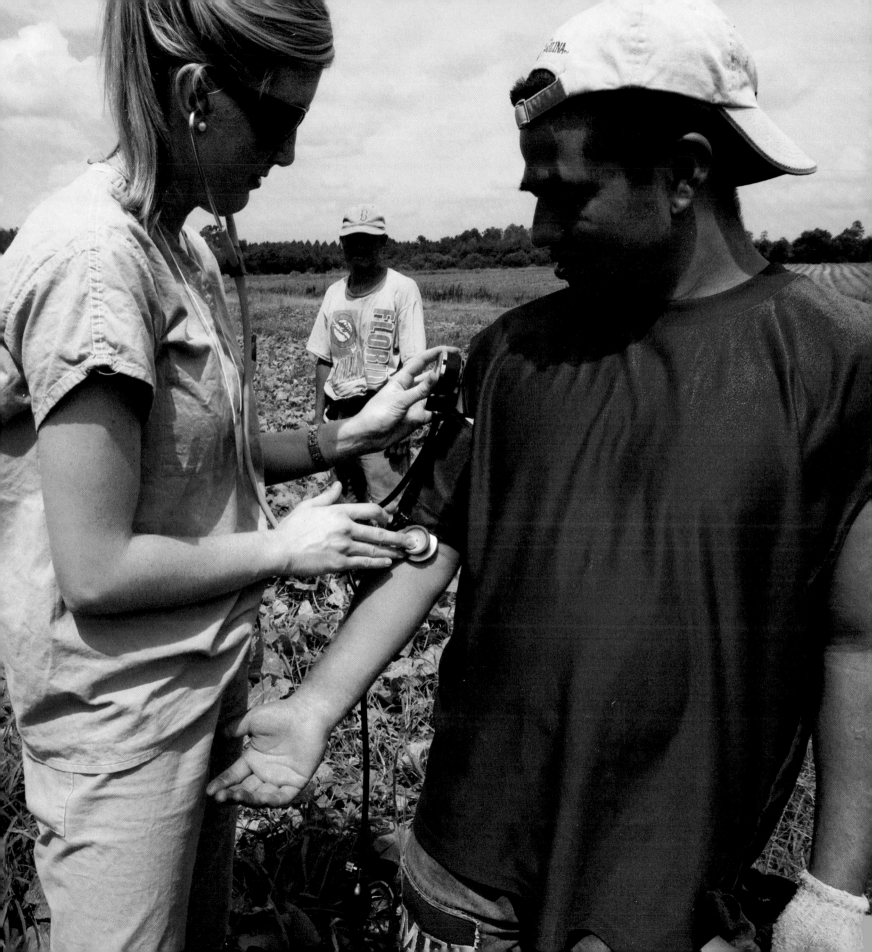

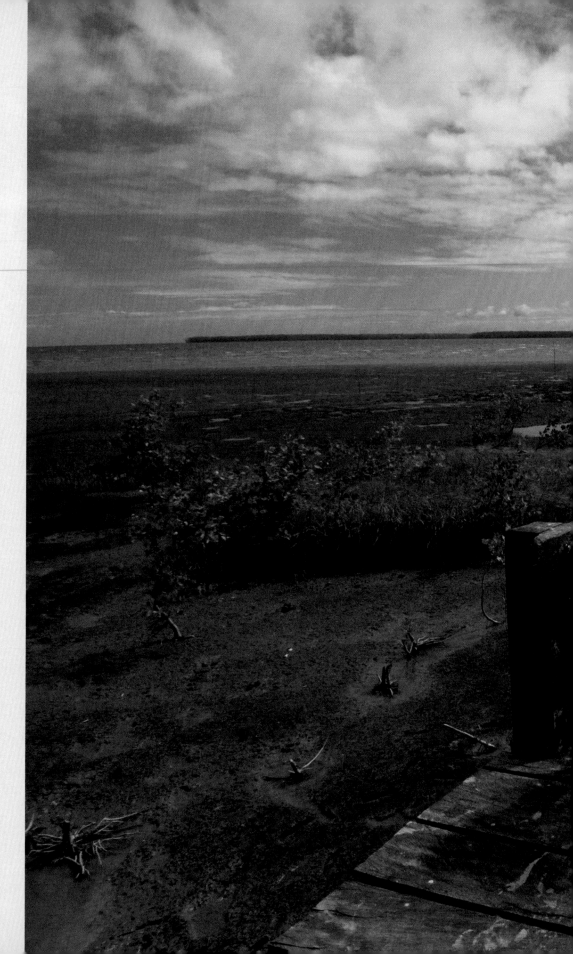

Malaria lurks in the swampy tidal flats of Venezuela, but field-research nurse Sister Isolena and a local "malaria hunter" are tracking signs of the invidious disease. Thanks to such diligence, malaria is no longer active in the area. Sister Isolena combines nursing with research, hoping to combat health problems in the homes of the poor and in the laboratory.

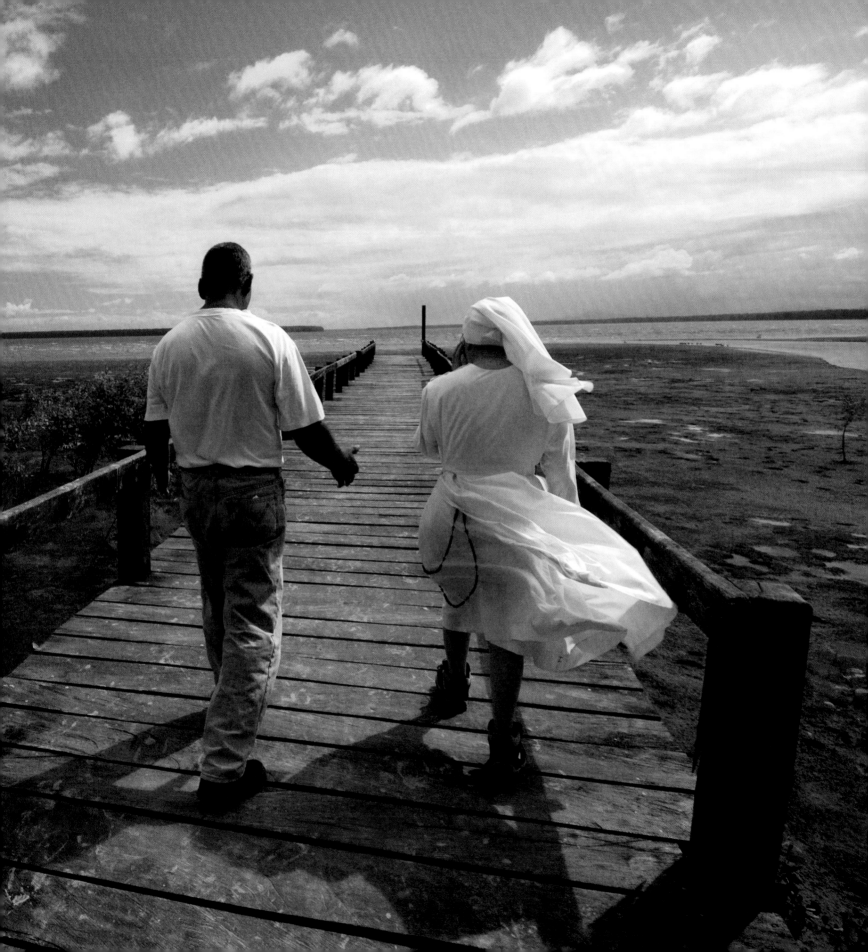

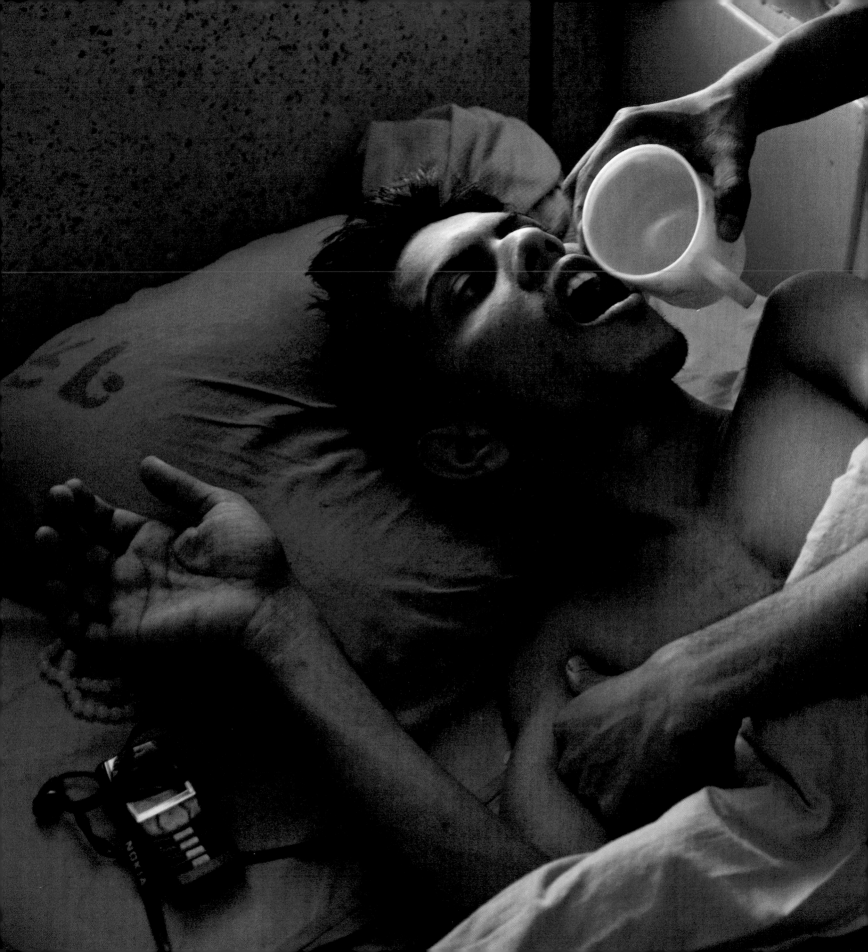

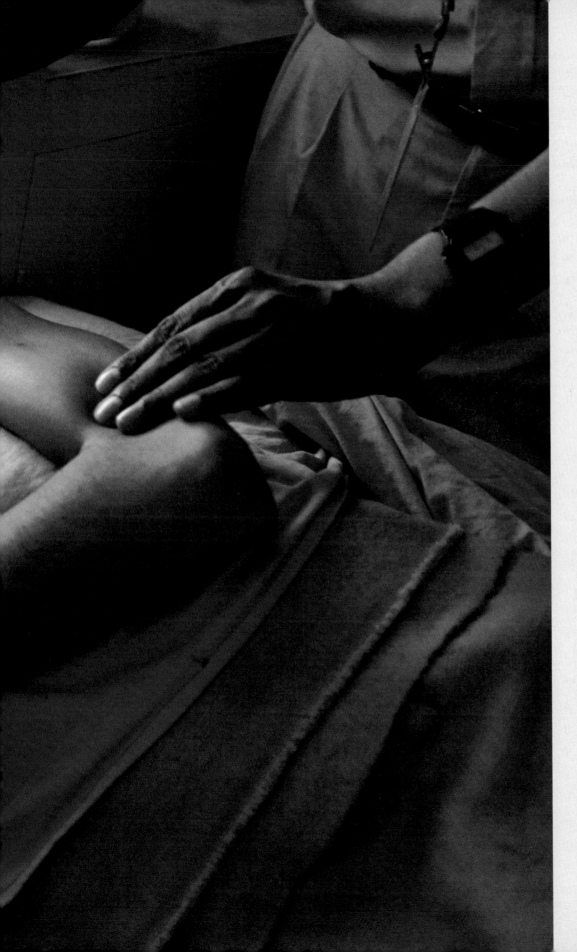

Kind hand with a cup, a nurse offers water to a patient at a rehabilitation center in rural Bangladesh. The center treats stroke victims and patients with spinal cord injuries, a common occurrence for the poor here, who spend long days in hard manual labor.

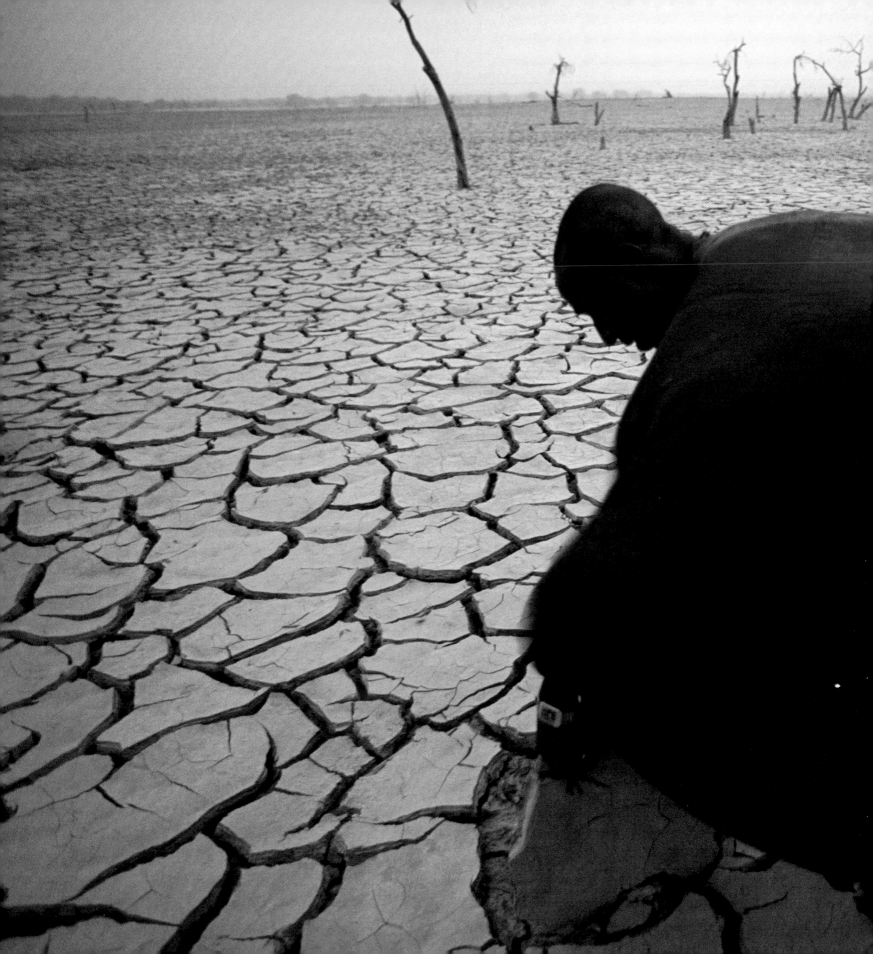

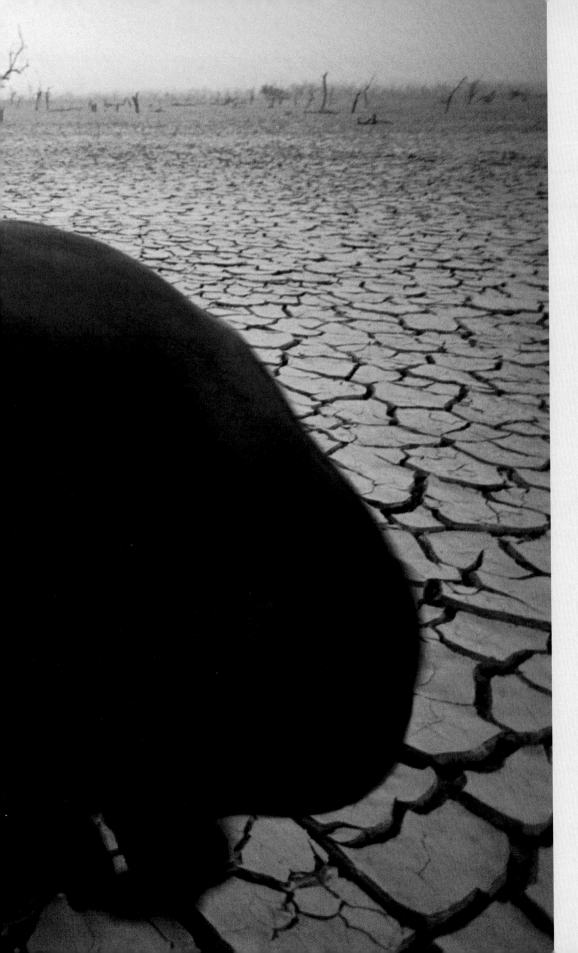

Waiting for the dry season to end has become an annual ordeal in much of Africa. This nurse in Mali is searching for any moisture that could be hidden in a dry lakebed, so that a poor rural village might find some respite from drought. Curse of much of the developing world, the lack of water not only results in dehydration but in poor hygiene and the resultant spread of disease.

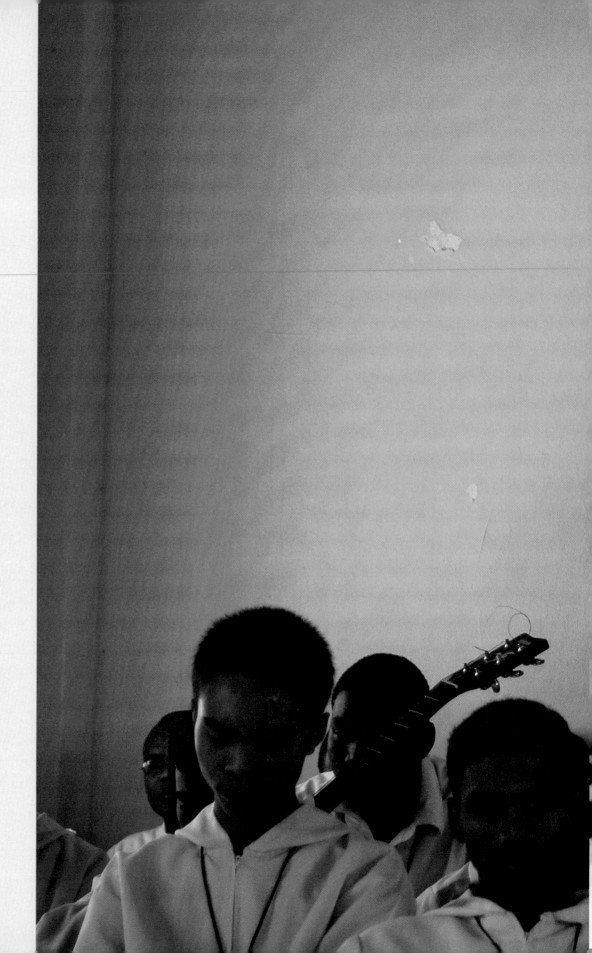

Inspired by their faith, Catholic Missionaries of the Poor in Kingston, Jamaica, welcome all those in need—the homeless and destitute, ill and troubled, young and old—providing them with basic health care and loving hands and hearts.

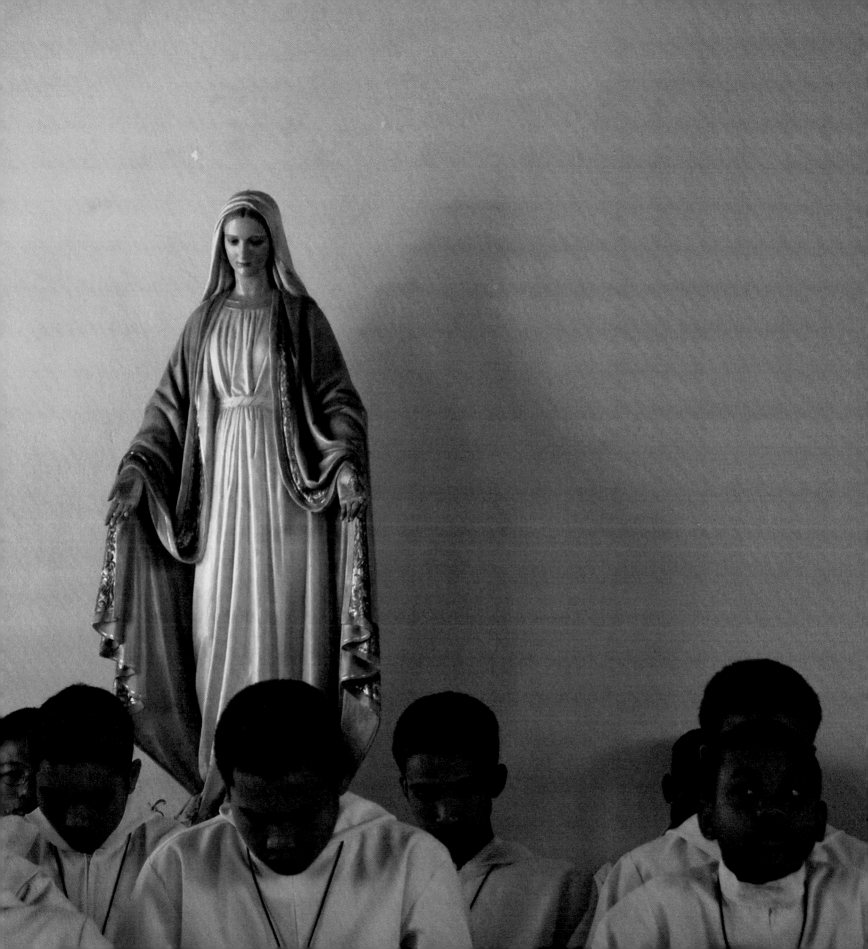

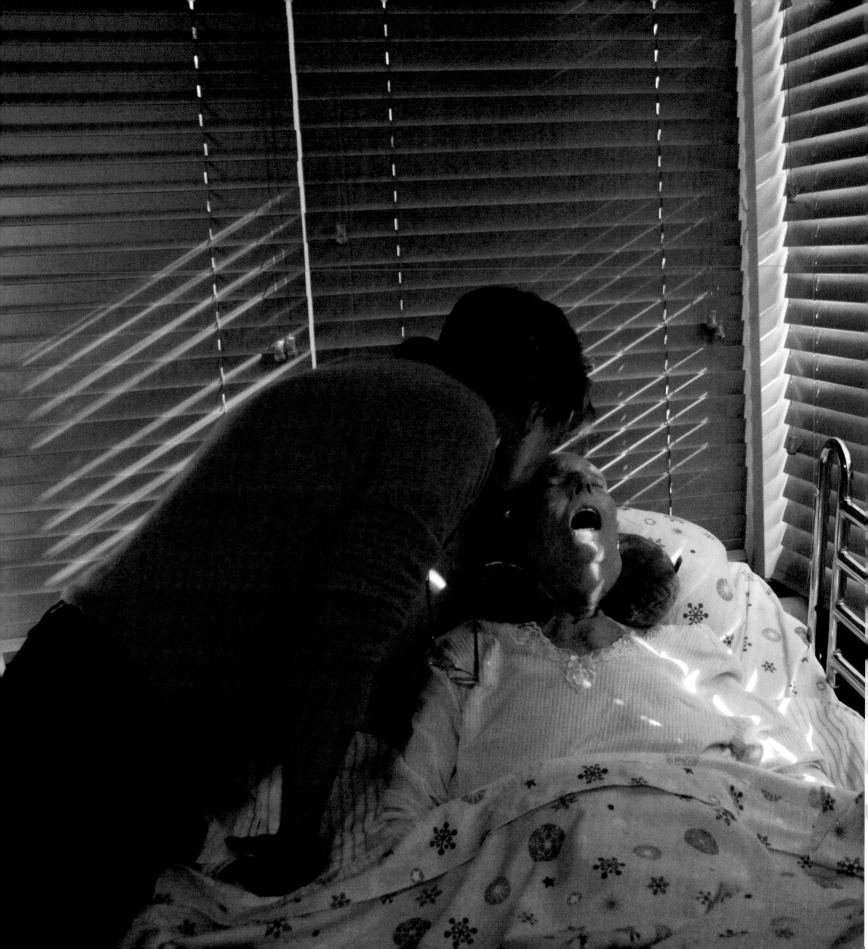

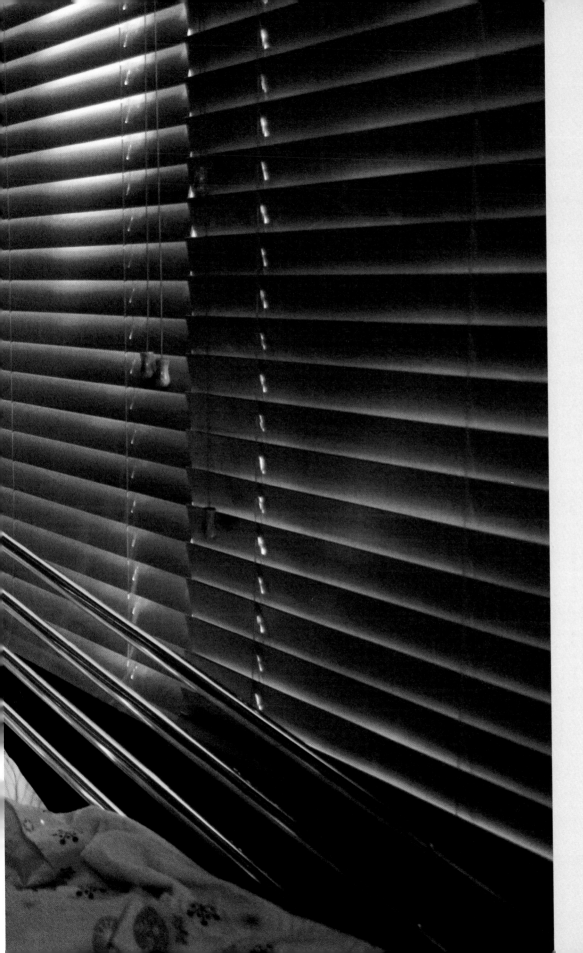

Nursing's final gift—helping to ease the pain of passing. This hospice nurse in Washington, D.C., tends a dying woman, offering palliative care and understanding to both her and her family and allowing her to spend her last days in her own home.

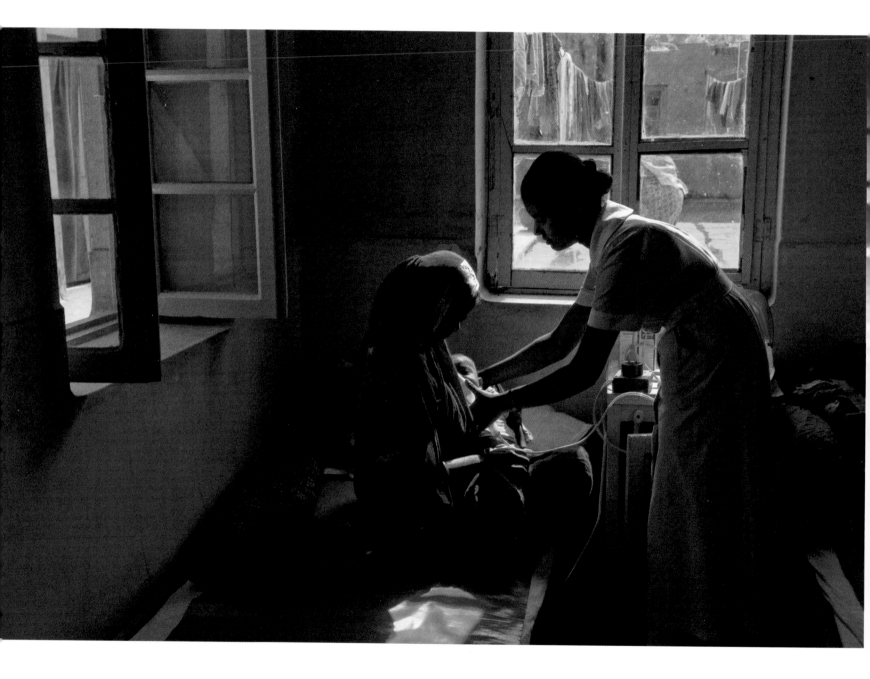

ONE   A TIMELESS LEGACY

In Bangladesh, where poverty is a way of life, the 750-bed Kumudini Hospital in Narayanganj is a god-send, offering free medical care to people from all over the country and training 250 nursing students each year. Kumudini students work their way through school, then continue as nurses at the hospital for two years after graduation.

The history of nursing has no beginning. Its origins lie in that most fundamental of human impulses: to care for those who are sick, frail, helpless, or in distress. There were nurses long before there was a profession of nursing, and the work they performed within the human community was so essential that it must have been taken for granted, as natural an act as nursing a baby or comforting a dying elder.

Even today, the work of nurses often remains invisible even where it is most essential. A village nurse in Sri Lanka walks miles to bring medicine to a remote outpost hit by cholera. A critical-care nurse in a pediatric intensive care unit takes a moment on a busy evening to hold a tiny, premature baby. A helicopter sweeps into the air as a military nurse gives a seriously wounded soldier a transfusion of blood. In the hills of Appalachia, a nurse midwife drives miles in the dark to assist in the birth of a young couple's first baby.

As nurses have done throughout the profession's long history, they give voice not through words but through actions. Their message is simple and profound: Those who are sick or in need deserve care and compassion, no matter who they are or where they may be.

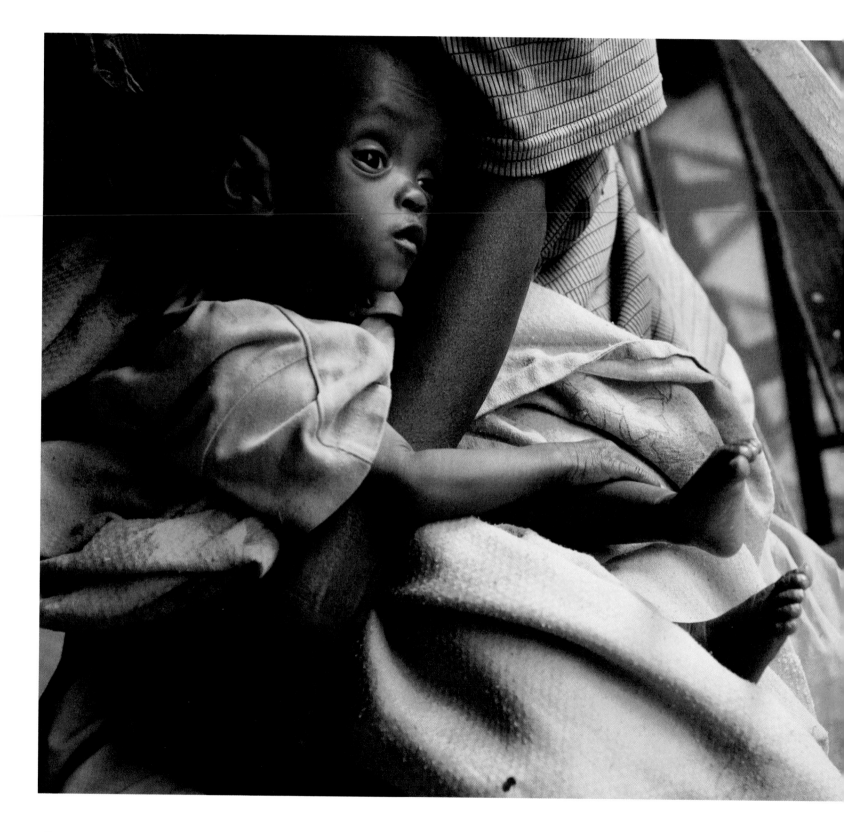

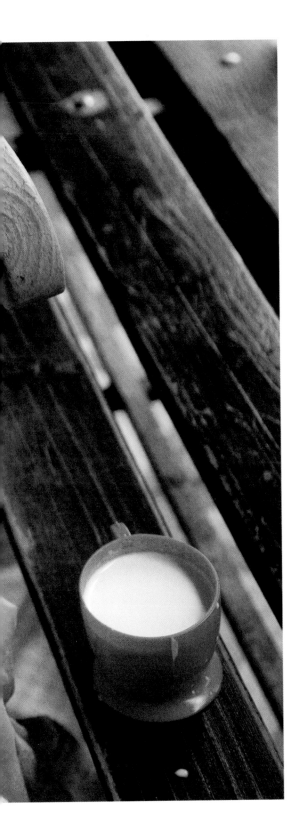

The word nursing comes from the Latin *nutrire*, "to nourish." Nursing has always been intimately associated with both midwifery and the nursing of infants—with helping to bring life into the world and with nurturing it. "So they sent their sister Rebekah on her way, along with her nurse and Abraham's servant and his men," the writer of Genesis recorded. A later passage conveys the esteem in which nurses were held. "Now Deborah, Rebekah's nurse, died and was buried under the oak below Bethel. So it was named 'oak of weeping.'"

Hippocrates is said to have created the first midwifery training program in Greece in the fifth century B.C. Long before then, of course, midwives were attending births—and sometimes speaking out movingly through their actions to defend the sanctity of life. When the pharaoh commanded that all sons born to Hebrew women be slaughtered, the Book of Exodus records the courageous defiance of the midwives who disobeyed him.

In many parts of the world, nursing evolved side by side with religion and the life of the spirit. The *Charaka Samhita,* one of the revered texts of ancient India, enumerates the traits of a fit nurse, who must be "of good behavior, distinguished for purity, possessed of cleverness and skill, imbued with kindness...skillful in waiting upon one that is ailing and never unwilling to do anything that may be ordered."

Feeding centers in much of sub-Saharan Africa are critical to keeping undernourished children alive. At this center in Harar, Ethiopia, children are fed a high-protein drink by the overworked nursing staff—only one nurse a shift for 25 to 50 young patients.

By the Middle Ages, Christian monasteries devoted to learning and prayer were taking on the work of nursing, which came to be considered not just a practice but a spiritual calling. In A.D. 529, St. Benedict declared that "the care of the sick is to be placed above and before every other duty, as if indeed Christ were being directly served by waiting on them." Many took up Benedict's call. In the sixth century, St. Radegunde established a hospice at Poitiers to care for lepers. St. Brigid founded a monastery at Kildare in Ireland, where she ministered to multitudes of the poor and infirm. Their work would be followed by generations of nurses associated with Christian orders, including the Augustinian nuns, the Sisters of Charity, and the Sisters of Mercy. Many hospitals in the U.S. still bear the name "Mercy," after the religious order that founded them.

Of all the early historical references to nursing, the most moving may be St. Jerome's eulogy, written in A.D. 399 upon the death of Fabiola, a matron in Rome who founded the first free Christian Hospital in that city. "How often have I seen her carrying in her arms these piteous, dirty, and revolting victims of the frightful malady! How often have I seen her wash wounds whose fetid water prevented everyone else from even looking at them! She fed the sick with her own hands, and revived the dying with small and frequent portions of nourishment . . . . If I had a hundred tongues in a clarion voice I could not enumerate the number of patients for whom Fabiola provided solace in the care."

It is telling that St. Jerome spoke on behalf of Fabiola and that we know her by her acts alone. Centuries would pass before nurses were able to raise their own voices on behalf of the art and science of

Nurses must be "of good behavior, distinguished for purity, possessed of cleverness and skill, imbued with kindness... skillful in waiting upon one that is ailing and never unwilling to do anything that may be ordered."

Charaka Samhita
Sacred Hindu text

nursing. With few exceptions, the ranks of nurses in most cultures have been dominated by women. Their contributions and their voices, like those of most women, were suppressed and sometimes forcibly silenced in male-dominated cultures, as they continue to be in some parts of the world. There are still places today where nurses are considered morally compromised because their work involves touching bodies.

But as women emerged from the shadows to demand recognition, nurses were at the forefront, speaking out for the importance of women's work in general and the mission of nursing in particular. And with what eloquence they spoke. "I come to present the strong claims of suffering humanity," a nurse named Dorothea Lynde Dix wrote in a pamphlet to the legislature of her home state, Massachusetts. The pamphlet was part of her nationwide crusade in the early 19th century to improve the scandalously cruel treatment of the mentally ill. "I come to place before the legislature of Massachusetts the condition of the miserable, the desolate, the outcast. I come as the advocate of helpless, forgotten, insane men and women; of beings sunk to a condition from which the unconcerned would start with real horror."

So powerful was her voice that when the Civil War erupted, Dix was named Superintendent of Army Nurses. In that role she distinguished herself by caring for both Union and Confederate wounded soldiers alike—part of a long tradition of nurses serving humanity during times of war and conflict. In the crowded wards of the injured and dying, she might well have glimpsed another nurse at work: Walt Whitman, the young nation's greatest poet, who spent much of the Civil War serving as a volunteer nurse ministering to wounded soldiers in Washington.

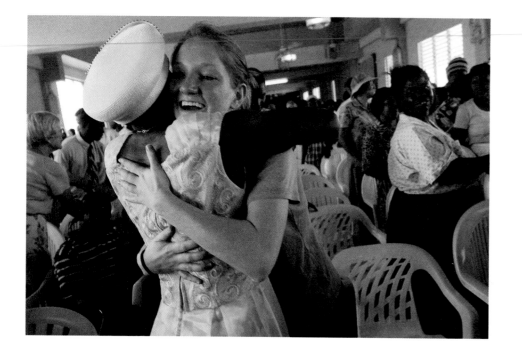

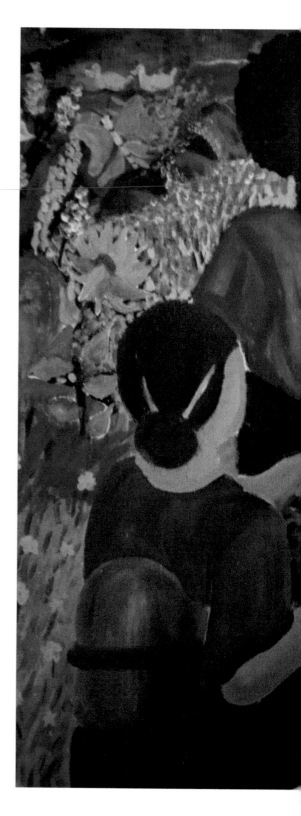

Hugs and smiles end a church service at one of the homes run by the
Missionaries of the Poor in Kingston, Jamaica, where Lydia Herron
(above) and other Emory University nursing students volunteer during
spring break. The missionaries take all those in need into their fold. Many
of the brothers—like the director, Brother Reynante (right)—are Filipinos
who came to Jamaica to serve God by serving "the poorest of the poor."

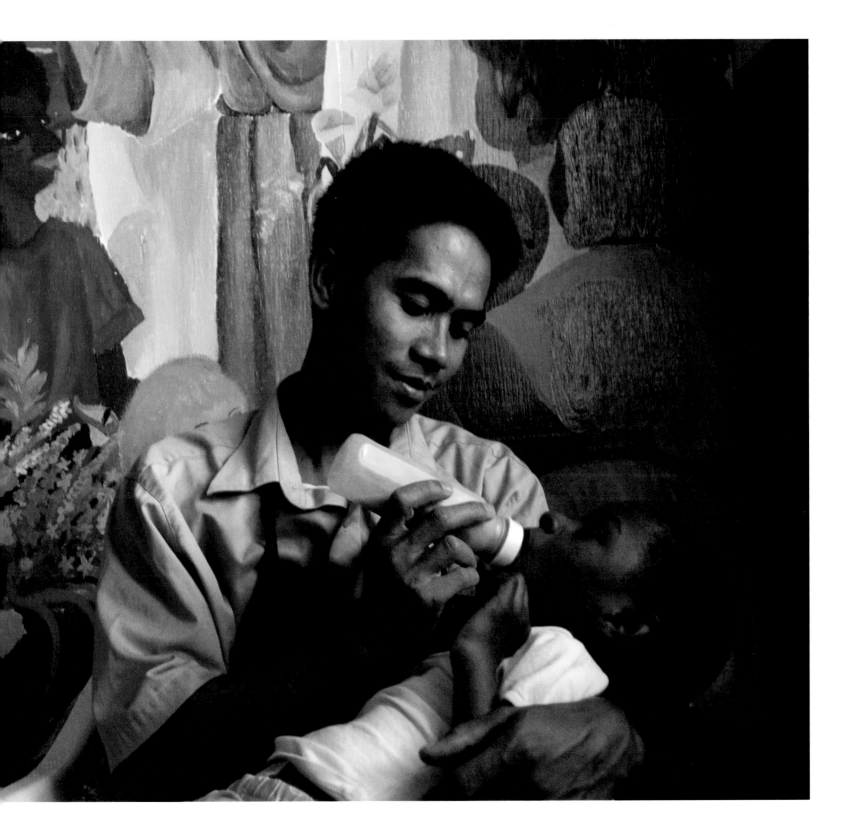

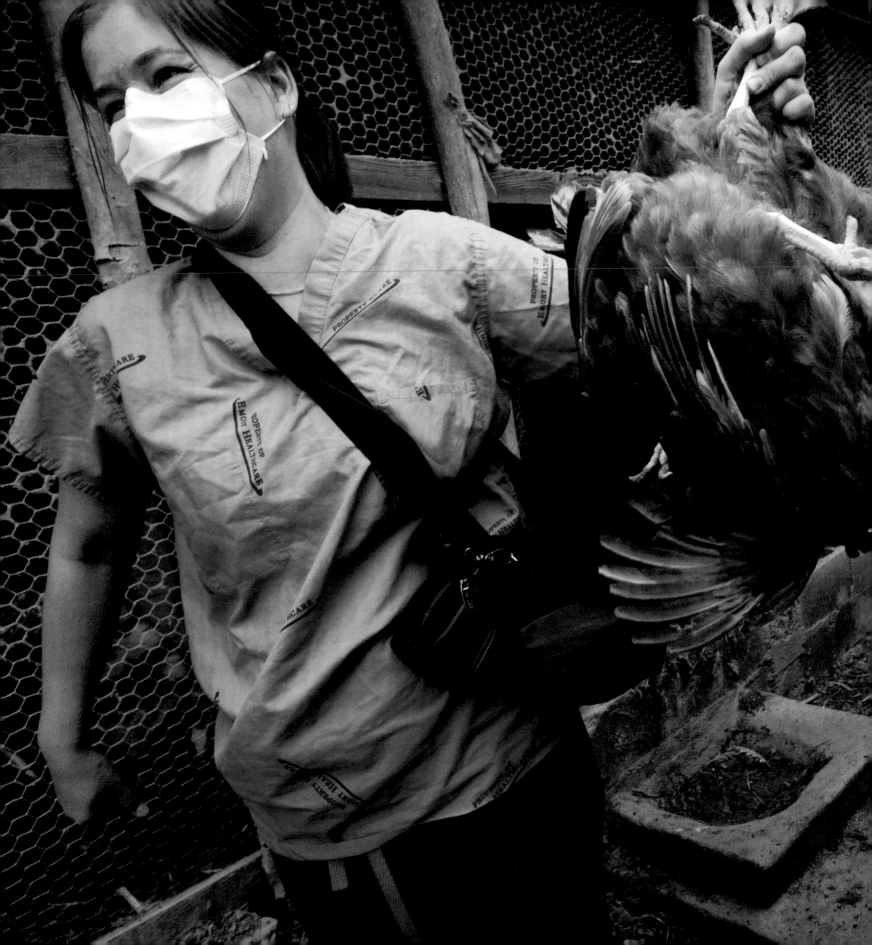

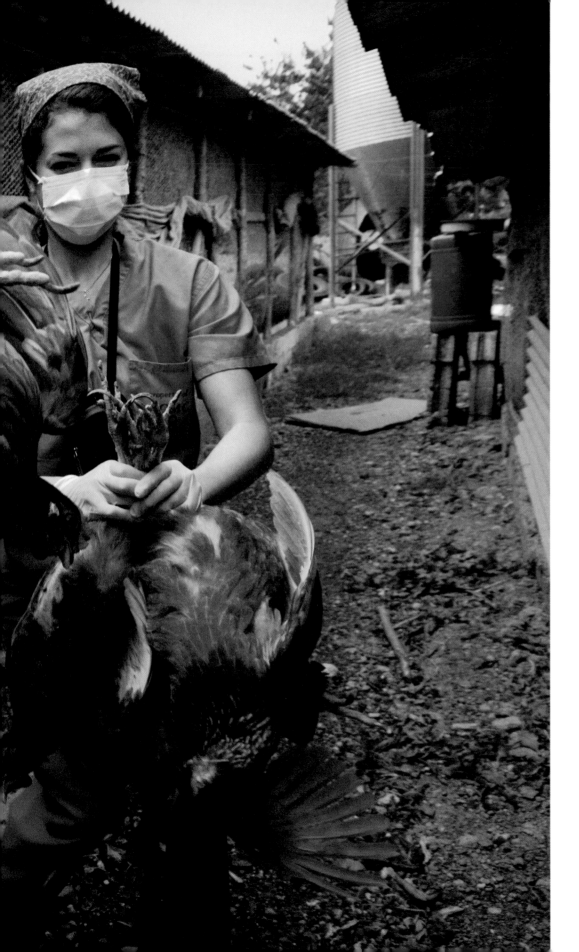

During their stay with the Missionaries of the Poor, Emory nursing students make an annual "chicken run" to a poultry farm outside Kingston. The chickens they collect and truck back to the city are handed out to needy Jamaicans, who gather in long lines for the passing of the poultry.

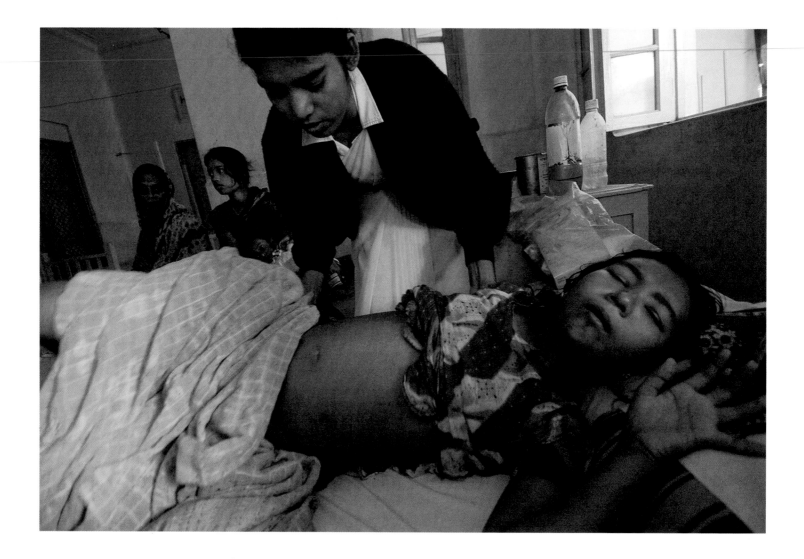

Outside Dhaka, Bangladeshi boys labor long hours in a brickmaking factory. Labor conditions, crushing poverty, and disease make a healthy life no more than a dream for many here. The young girl (left) has come to Kumudini Hospital with pain, fever, and a swollen abdomen; a nursing student is helping assess her condition.

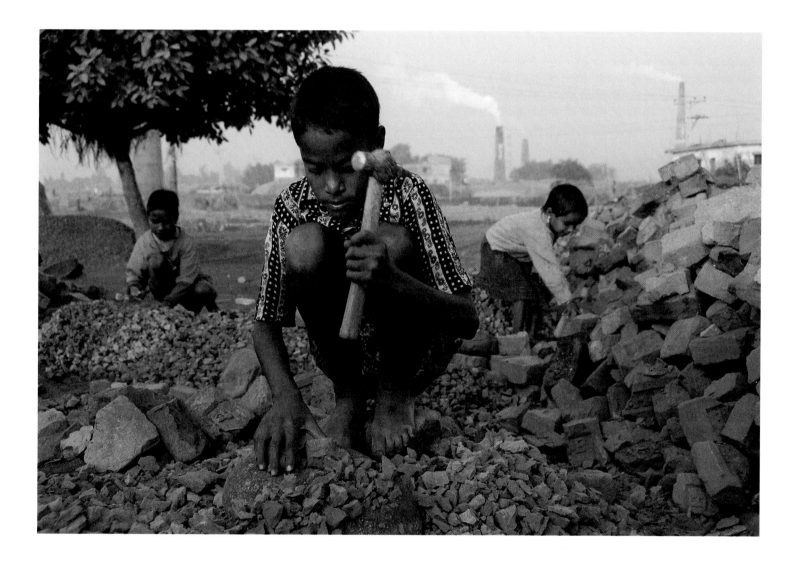

In "The Wound-Dresser," he turned the brutal horrors of war and the sometimes harrowing work of nursing into enduring poetry.

Bearing the bandages, water and sponge,
Straight and swift to my wounded I go,
Where they lie on the ground after the battle brought in,
Where their priceless blood reddens the grass, the ground...

From the stump of the arm, the amputated hand,
I undo the clotted lint, remove the slough,
Wash off the matter and blood,
Back on his pillow the soldier bends with
Curv'd neck and side falling head,
His eyes are closed, his face is pale, he
Dares not look on the bloody stump,
And has not yet look'd on it.

Whitman almost certainly knew the reputation of another nurse working in Britain, who had rushed to the cause of injured soldiers during the Crimean War and who would go on to found the modern profession of nursing. "Nursing is not an adventure, as some have now supposed," she wrote late in her life. "It is a very serious, delightful thing, like life, requiring training, experience, devotion not by fits and starts, patience, a power of accumulating, instead of losing—all these things."

The words are Florence Nightingale's, written in 1897. Nightingale made so many contributions to the art and science of nursing, and spoke

> "Nursing is not an adventure.... It is a very serious, delightful thing, like life, requiring training, experience, devotion...a power of accumulating, instead of losing—all these things."
>
> *Florence Nightingale*

out on so many subjects, that even today the full extent of her contribution is only beginning to be understood. She reformed Britain's army medical system, argued for the importance of sanitation and good diet, created plans for hospitals designed to promote healing, and started the Nightingale Training School for Nurses in London; the first modern secular school of nursing, it would spread its influence around the world. In the course of her lifetime she wrote over a hundred books and reports, as well as tens of thousands of letters, including the largest single personal collection of letters in the British Library.

Nightingale inspired generations of nursing students. She spoke up for the dispossessed and demanded that those in power try to end unnecessary suffering. She understood that the social and physical environments people live in—the conditions of their homes and neighborhoods, their access to adequate food and water—are critical to health. Indeed, she gave voice to a new idea: that nursing's mission involved not only caring for the individual but for the community and society at large. Enlightened social policies, she came to understand, were as essential to improving health as the most dedicated work at the bedside, a powerful idea that remains an essential part of nursing. At the same time, Nightingale never stopped advancing the art and science of nursing at the bedside, promoting a quest for new knowledge and expertise that remains a driving force in nursing to this day.

Nightingale's story is well known. That of another nurse working as her contemporary is less familiar. Mary Seacole, born in Kingston, Jamaica, in 1805, was the daughter of a Scottish soldier and a Jamaican mother. She learned the traditional medicine of the Caribbean and

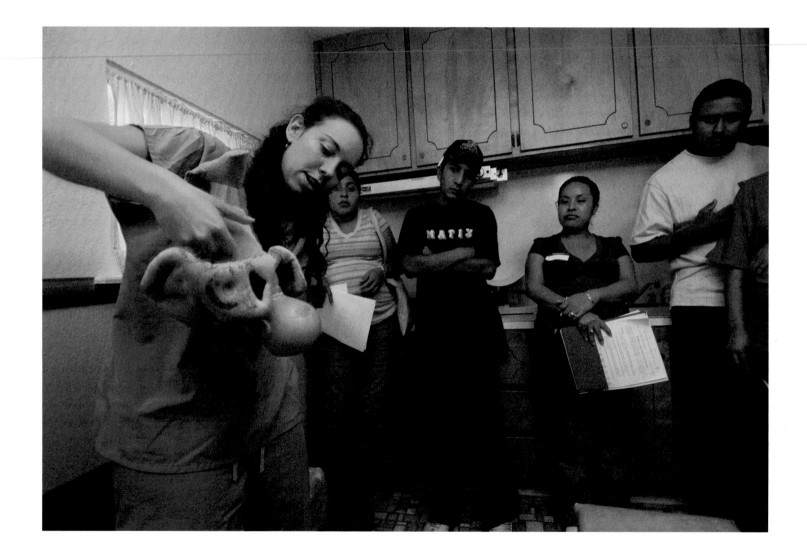

Nurses and nurse midwives from across the U.S. volunteer a year or more of their time to the Holy Family Birth Center in Weslaco, Texas. Classes at the center (left) help expectant mothers and fathers prepare for all aspects of parenting—from prenatal nutrition to birth to infant care. When the moment arrives, nurse midwives are on hand (below) to help bring the baby into the world.

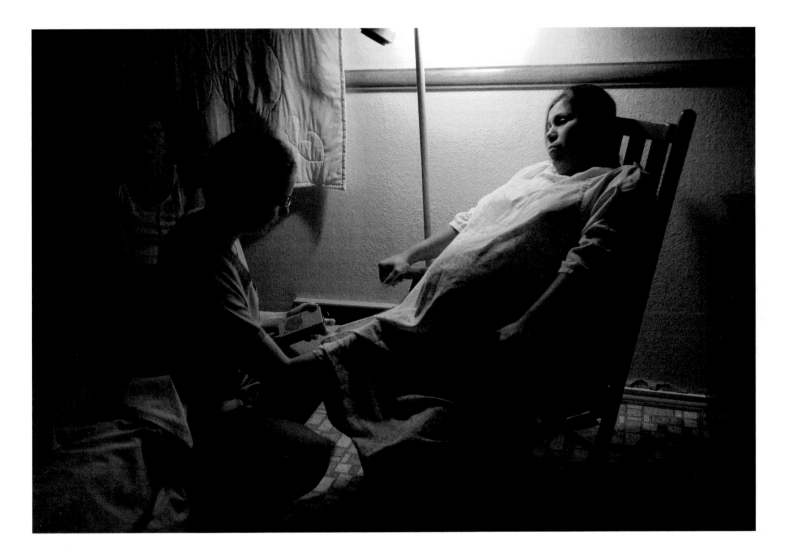

Africa from her mother, a "doctress" who often treated European soldiers and sailors suffering from tropical illnesses, sometimes even assisting at the British army hospital in Jamaica. Seacole eventually traveled around the Caribbean, made the long passage to England several times, and worked as a nurse in Panama, where she gained experience in treating cholera patients.

In 1854, learning that Florence Nightingale was assembling a team of nurses to treat wounded British soldiers in the Crimea, Seacole traveled at her own expense to London to volunteer. She was turned down by British authorities there—not for lack of experience but because she was of mixed race. Undaunted, she paid her own way to the Crimea and set up a small hotel where she treated sick and injured soldiers. On one occasion she was wounded herself while ministering to troops under fire.

"She is always in attendance near the battle-field to aid the wounded and has earned many a poor fellow's blessing," a correspondent with the *London Times* wrote in September 1855. Seacole wrote about her intrepid life in *Wonderful Adventures of Mrs. Seacole in Many Lands.* Published in 1857, it was the first autobiography ever written by a black woman in Britain.

While Seacole was honored in her lifetime, her contribution was soon largely forgotten—a reminder of how deeply sexism, racism, and other forms of discrimination influence the historical record. As the novelist Salman Rushdie wrote, "See, here is Mary Seacole, who did as much in the Crimea as another magic-lamping lady, but, being dark, could scarce be seen for the flame of Florence's candle . . . ."

With health care ever more expensive in the U.S., school nurses have taken on a greater role in family health. A pioneering program in Silver Spring, Maryland, allows the whole family to receive check-ups from a nurse practitioner, at left, while the school nurse, at right, is always on hand for daily needs.

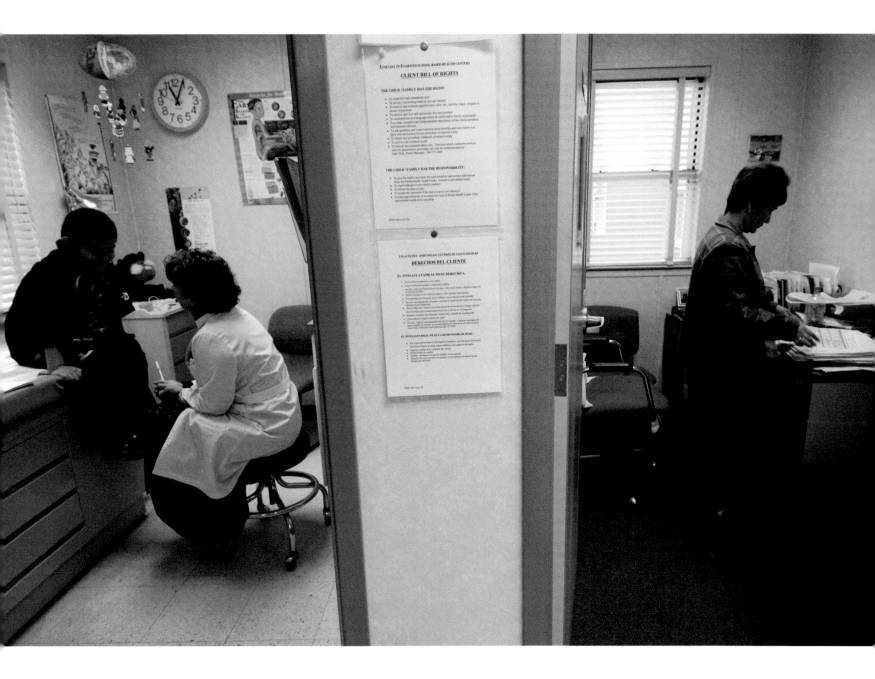

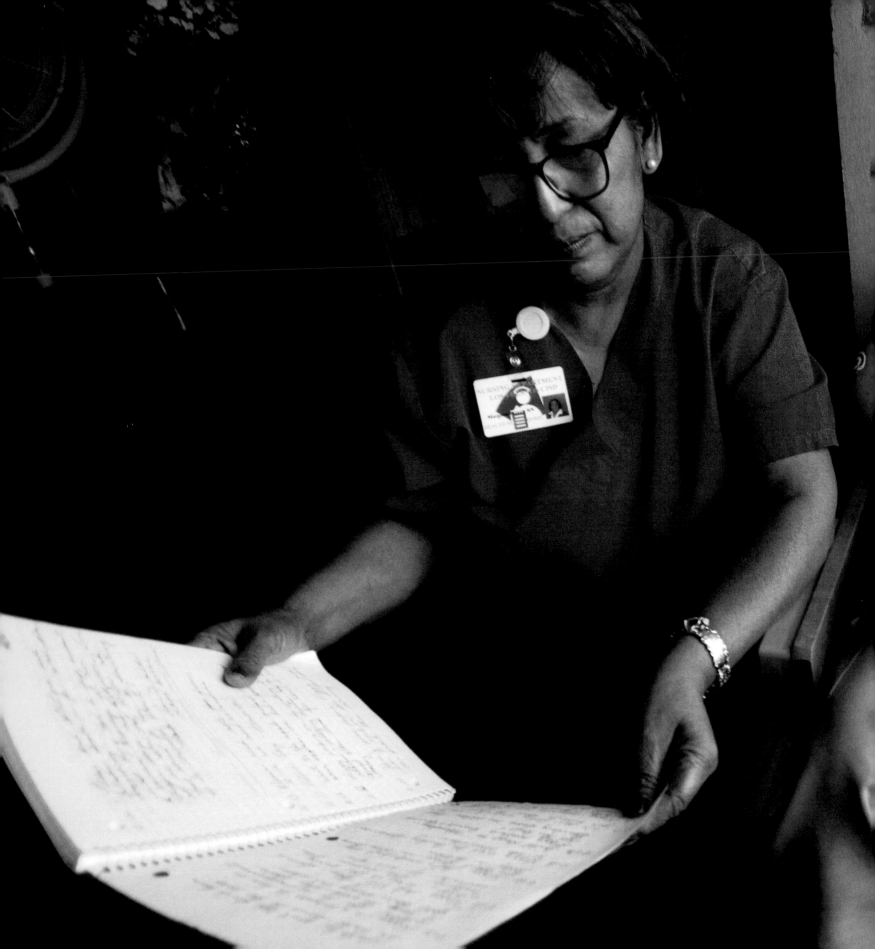

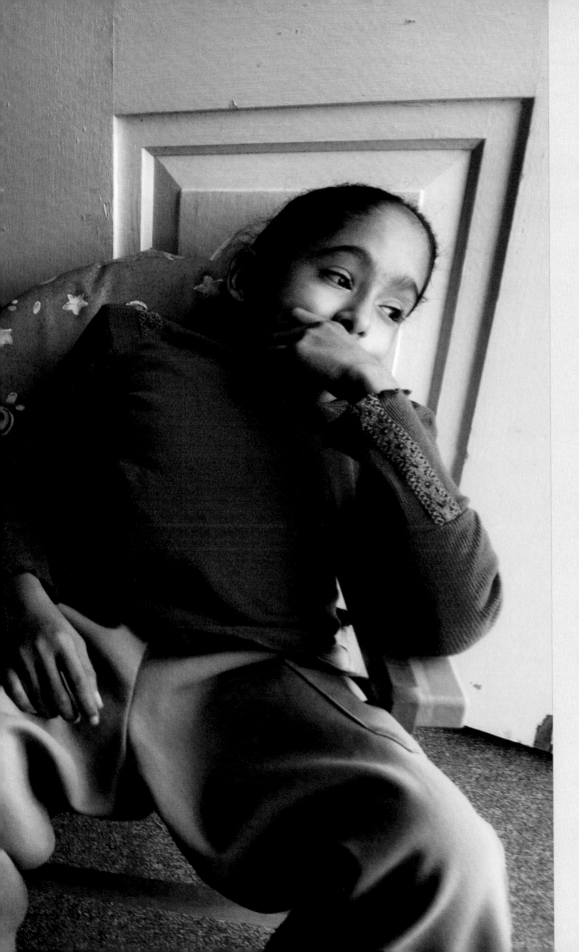

HEALTH ANGEL

Lizzy Garcia, on the right, has done a lot of living in her short life. She's learned to cope with spina bifida, a congenital malformation of her spinal cord that has left her wheelchair-bound. And she's learned to adjust to an annual move between her winter home in Cameron County, Texas, and the summer fields of northern states, as her father, a migrant worker, moves his family with the seasons. But every year when she returns to Texas,

On a visit to Lizzy's home, nurse and family friend Maggie Perez runs a careful but affectionate eye over the girl's schoolwork.

Lizzy is greeted by her friend, Maggie Perez. Once Lizzy's school nurse, Maggie has long been a friend of the Garcia family. She knew the family before Lizzy was born, when the parents and older children were living in a bus on land they managed to buy.

Today, through hard work and diligence, the Garcias own their own home here. And Maggie has become coordinator for health services in the county, supervising a number of nurses in school clinics and other facilities. But despite her many responsibilities, Maggie remains Lizzie's self-appointed health angel.

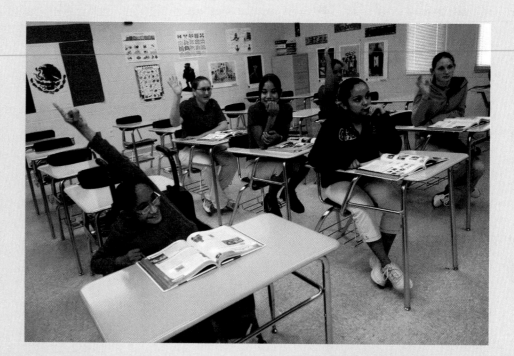

An enthusiastic student, Lizzy enjoys her days at Liberty Memorial Middle School, where she's in classes with teenage girls her own age. In the school clinic, nurse Kathryn Hale (below) catheterizes Lizzy and takes care of other daily health issues resulting from her condition.

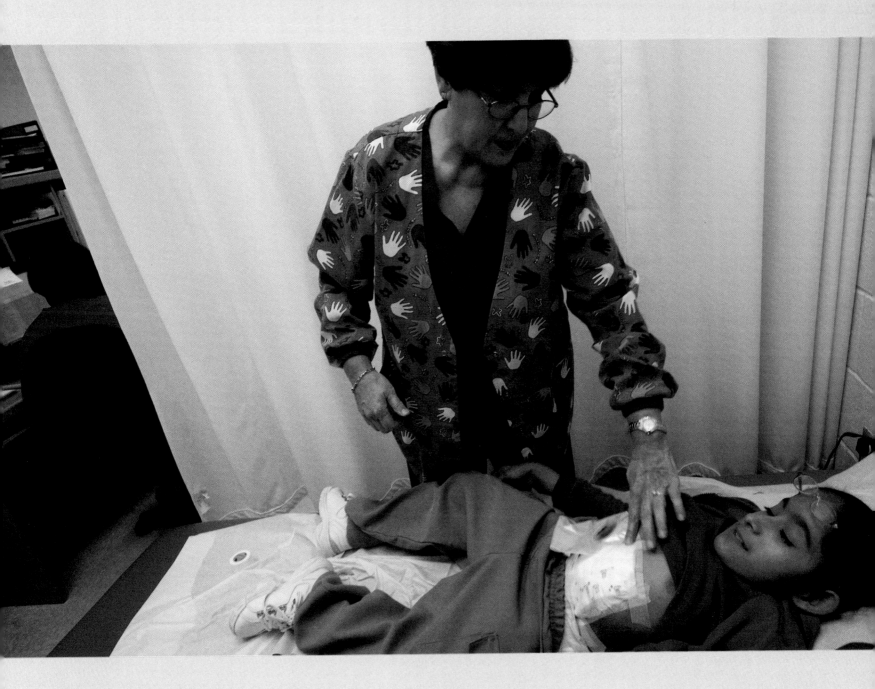

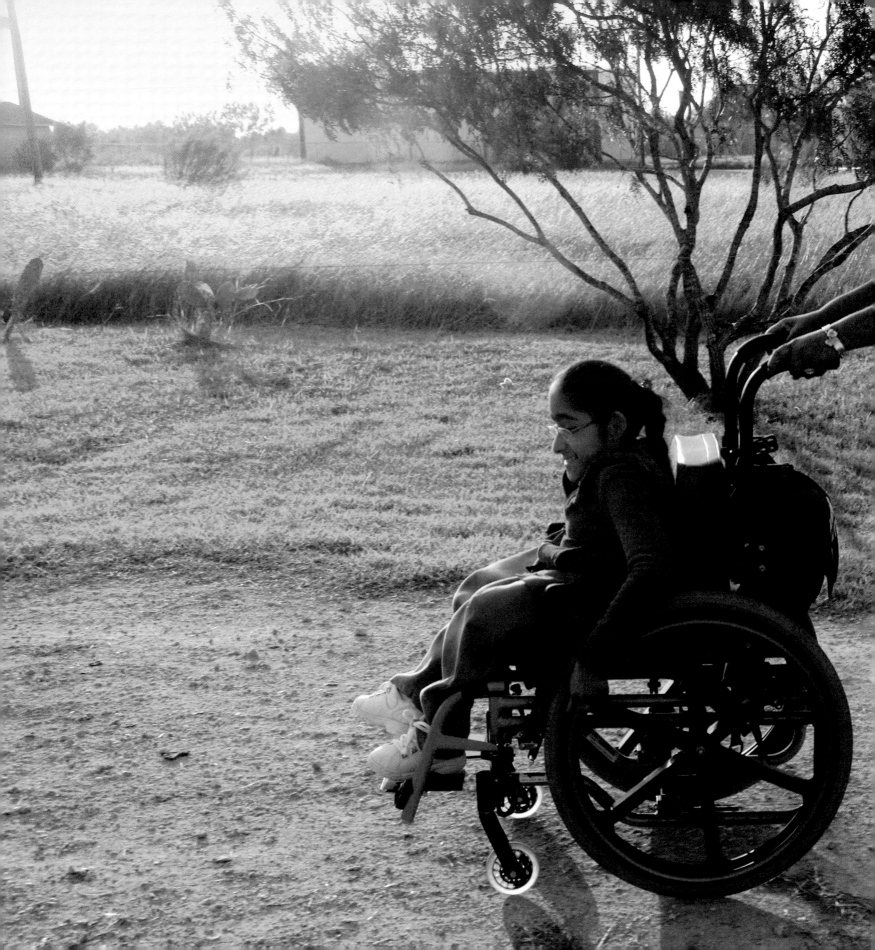

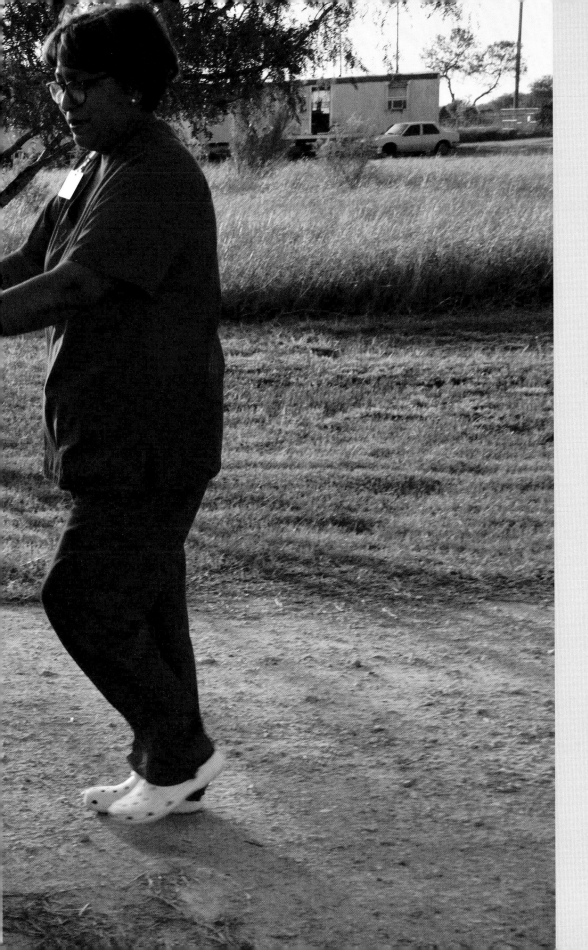

After-school stroll: Escaping her busy schedule, Maggie occasionally finds time to walk Lizzy from the school bus stop to her home. Because Lizzy's family is often on the move, her health needs could become lost among too many providers. But Maggie keeps close track of Lizzy's problems and progress throughout the year.

TO BE SURE, SEACOLE HERSELF RAILED AGAINST RACISM. WHEN AN AMERICAN who was supposedly honoring her at a dinner said, "If we could bleach her by any means we would . . . and thus make her acceptable in any company as she deserves to be," she shot back that she would be happy to have a complexion "as dark as any nigger's" and instead suggested "the general reformation of American manners."

Seacole would be joined by a long tradition of nurses crusading to end not only racism but all forms of discrimination. The progress of nursing has been intimately connected with the steady march of social justice, advocating for the rights of women, minorities, the poor and the dispossessed. The nurses' motives have been at once high-minded and pragmatic. Only when the vast inequalities that separate people are bridged can nursing truly fulfill its mission of providing care to everyone, regardless of who they are—male or female, of high class or low, rich or poor.

Indeed, many nurses have worked to bridge the economic gap, to bear witness to the harsh inequalities in the world and their consequences. "That morning's experience was a baptism by fire," an American nurse named Lillian D. Wald would write in the early 1900s, recalling the experience of being led by a little girl whose mother was ailing through the appalling squalor of New York's Lower East Side. Here, new immigrants to the city lived in conditions of almost unspeakable filth, poverty, and disease. "To my inexperience it seemed certain that conditions such as these were allowed because people did not know; and for me there was a challenge to know and to tell," Wald wrote, "and I rejoiced that I had a training in the care of the sick that in itself would give me an organic relationship to the neighborhood in which this awakening had come."

> "Nursing is love in action, and there is no finer manifestation of it than the care of the poor and disabled in their own homes."
>
> *Lillian Wald*

To know and to tell. That powerful phrase perfectly conveys nursing's mission to witness and speak for those who have no voice. Galvanized by the suffering she'd seen, Wald went on to found the Henry Street Settlement and the Visiting Nurse Service of New York. Under her guidance, a small staff of ten nurses began visiting the poor and forgotten in their homes, giving rise to the practice of home-care nursing. By 1916, 250 nurses in New York were caring for some 1,300 patients a day. Wald lobbied tirelessly for the creation of the Federal Children's Bureau, whose mission was to protect children from abuse and child labor. Run mostly by women, the agency helped states provide health care services for children and their mothers. According to University of Virginia nursing historian Barbara Brodie, the Children's Bureau was the forerunner of Title 5 of the Social Security Act, as well as Medicare and Medicaid.

Like Florence Nightingale, Wald is honored not only in the field of nursing but in other disciplines as well. Nightingale is celebrated for her pioneering use of biostatistics and for understanding the importance of hygiene in preventing infectious disease. Wald launched the field of social work in America and crusaded for civil rights. That work in areas outside of nursing exemplifies another feature of the profession: that the form of nursing often follows function. Throughout history, nurses have taken up whatever tools worked—whether a rag soaked in carbolic acid or a protest banner—to care for those in need. "Nursing," Lillian Wald wrote, "is love in action, and there is no finer manifestation of it than the care of the poor and disabled in their own homes."

Around the world, others took up Wald's cause. One was a woman from a distinguished Kentucky family. Mary Breckenridge had suffered personal tragedy and loss herself and turned to nursing and midwifery as a way to help others in need. In the 1920s, she rode on horseback through the rugged hills of eastern Kentucky, visiting small hamlets with few roads and virtually no medical care, where women gave birth to an average of nine children and where shockingly high numbers of them died in childbirth. Deeply troubled by what she saw, Breckenridge went on to found the Frontier Nursing Service. Many of the midwives she organized had been trained in England, as she had been, at the schools Nightingale had created. Now they were traveling on horse and foot across an area of 700 square miles, offering prenatal and childbirth care in the poorest and most remote areas of Kentucky. Breckenridge, who is credited with bringing midwifery to the United States, honored the dignity of those she served in her characteristically humble way. "I am not trying to help them," she insisted. "We and they are cooperating . . . they are fine, intelligent citizens."

In words like these, nursing speaks of more than simple compassion. It declares the essential dignity of every person. The work of nursing is grounded in harsh physical realities. Nurses, after all, care for bodies. They know the worst indignities that can be visited upon flesh and bone. But nurses also defend the essential dignity of people simply by caring for them and by honoring the life of the spirit. Indeed, few professions encompass so much of what it is to be human as does nursing.

Today's nurses often speak of themselves as patient advocates—a role that has become critically important in the labyrinthine, impersonal, and sometimes cruel maze of modern health care. Nurses are that, but they are much more besides. In the increasingly technological world of

A young nurse midwife-in-training proudly shows off her own baby at the Frontier School of Midwifery & Family Nursing, the Kentucky institution founded by Mary Breckenridge in the 1920s. Students at FSMFN do most of their academic training online and in their own communities, but they also come to Hyden, Kentucky, periodically for training, sharing, and bonding.

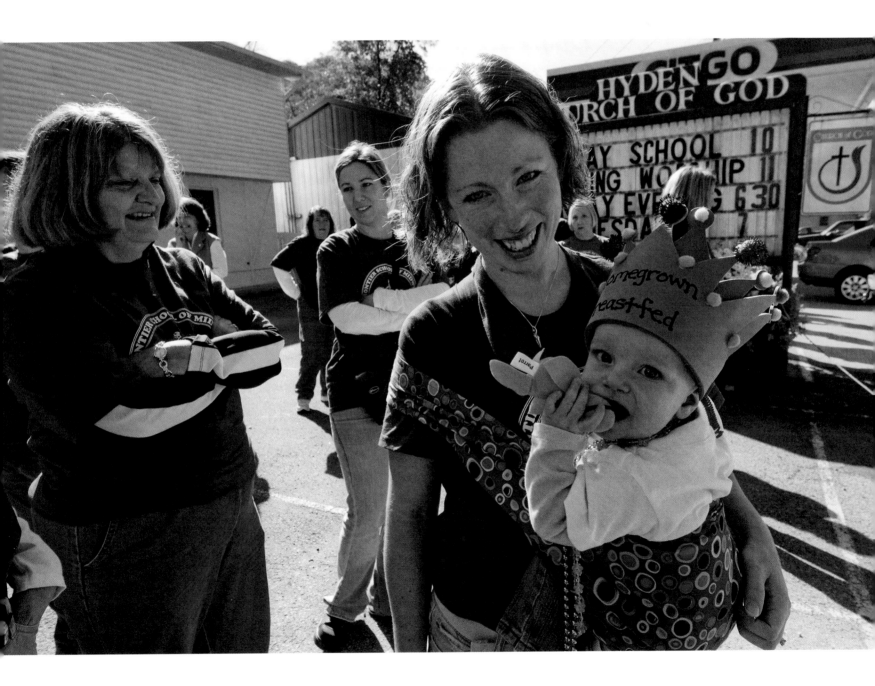

A community of care: At a convent in Caracas, Venezuela, nuns who serve as nurses find solace in their own time of need. Here, Sister Isolena, at right—at 80 still a dynamic field-research nurse—lends support to an aging fellow nun.

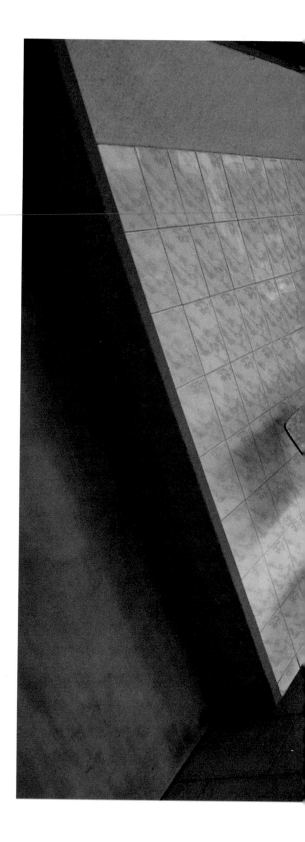

modern medicine, nurses preserve the human touch. They are advocates for whole and healthy families, for communities where children are safe and sheltered, where the frail elderly can live with dignity, and where people, free of fear and discrimination, can achieve their full human potential. Nurses often become part of the community in order to do their work. Recalling her experiences working after the revolution in her home country, Cuban-born nurse Nancy Olivera perfectly captured the challenge. "When I knocked on a door, the farmers would close it . . . . But when they didn't let me in, I would go around to the back door and insist. I got to know them. I ate with them and little by little taught them better hygiene."

By providing even the most basic care—indeed, simply by caring—nurses can create order and a sense of community, even in the most extreme and violent settings. "I still remember the day we had to evacuate the town of Muhajeria where we'd been working," recalled Elizabeth Liszt, a nurse for Doctors Without Borders, the international medical relief organization. For almost a year she had been helping treat sick and wounded refugees in the Sudan and Chad. "We had 1,200 children in the feeding center who were dependent on us for food, and we were seeing 120 people in the clinic every day."

Despite increasing danger, Liszt and a small staff kept working until they were ordered to leave. She never had any second thoughts. "I became a nurse because this is the kind of work I want to do," she said. When the order finally came to evacuate, Liszt could see villages burning. "These were people we knew. We mourned and cried so many tears. And then we said, 'Okay, that's enough. Let's get out there and try to do something.'"

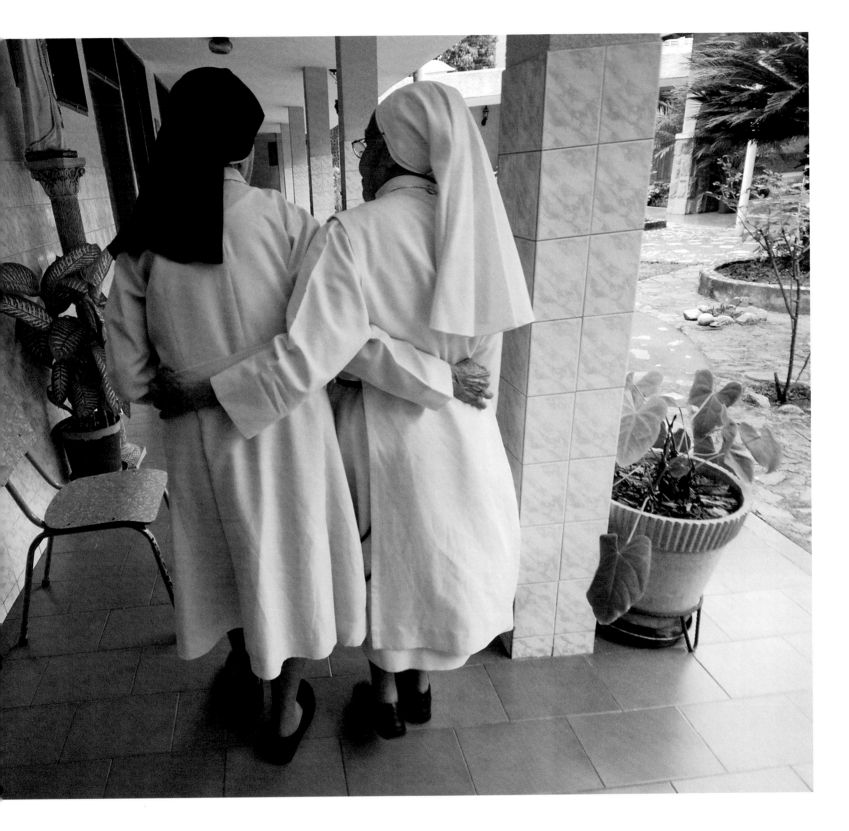

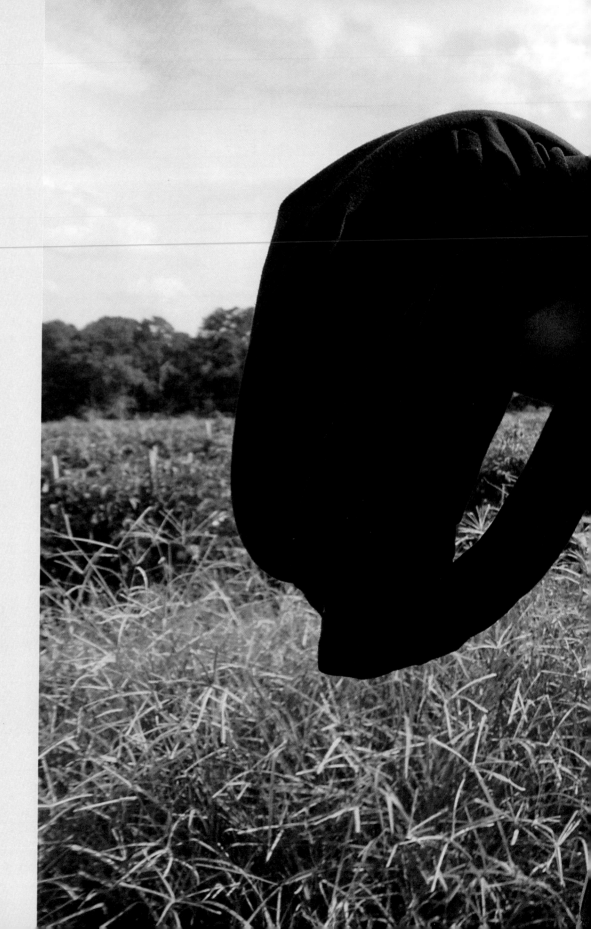

KEEPING MIGRANT FAMILIES HEALTHY

Each year tens of thousands of migrant workers and their families descend on southwest Georgia to harvest and package fruits, vegetables, tobacco. Every day's wage is important, so few can take time off for their own health care or that of their children.

A dozen years ago, health professionals in Georgia realized this

On a break from the hot, hard hours in the fields, a migrant worker has his blood pressure taken by a student nurse volunteering with the Farm Worker Family Health Program.

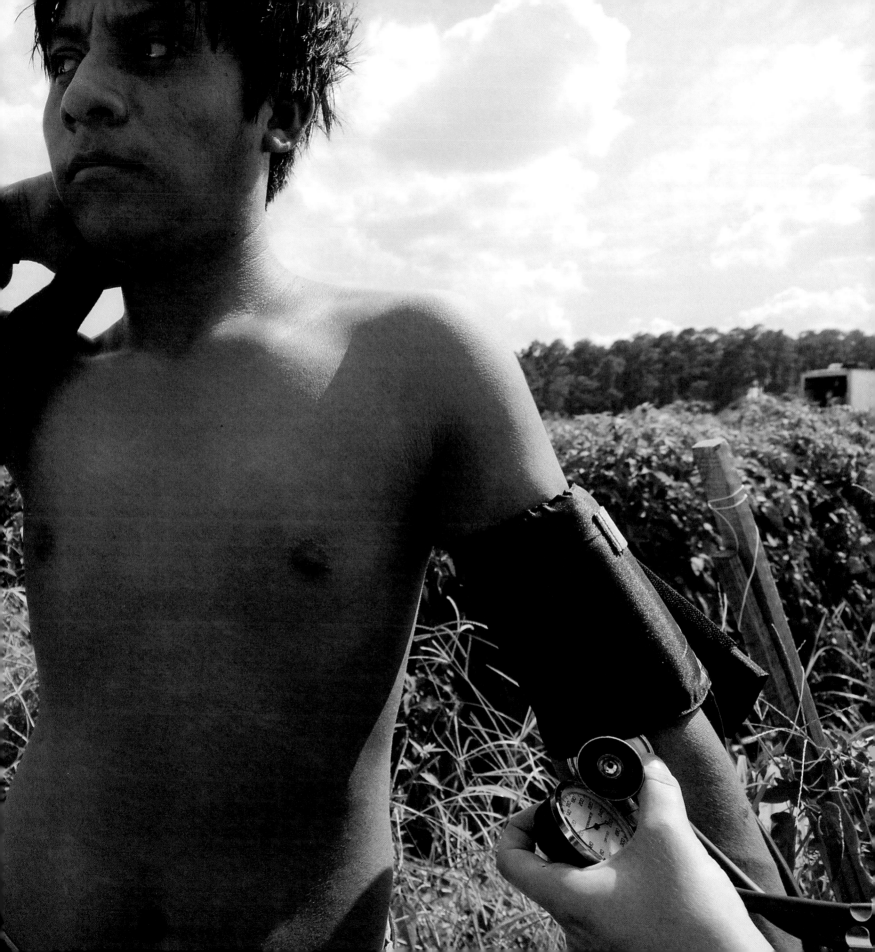

and organized what is now the Farm Worker Family Health Program. Every June volunteers from Emory University's Nell Hodgson Woodruff School of Nursing and from other institutions spend two weeks in the fields, schools, and clinics around Moultrie, Georgia, offering free health and dental care to people who otherwise would receive little—or none at all.

Mornings, nursing students and other health volunteers fan out to an area school and clinic, to do medical, developmental, and psychological evaluations on the children of migrant families. Evenings, the volunteers focus on the farms, where workers are coming off a day in the fields and finally have time for health evaluations and treatment of the aches and pains that come

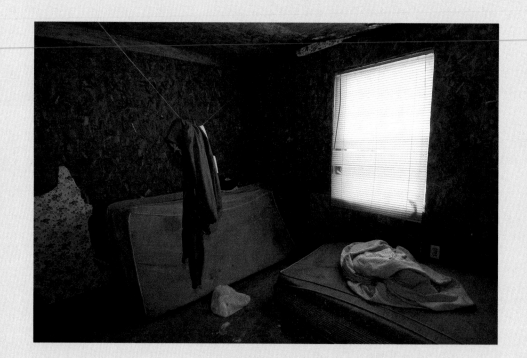

Some employers offer migrants shelters that are no more than hovels (left). Harsh conditions and the constant moving are hard on families, particularly kids, whose education and health can suffer. But repeat volunteers with the Farm Worker Family Health Program often form friendships (below) with parents and kids that are renewed year after year.

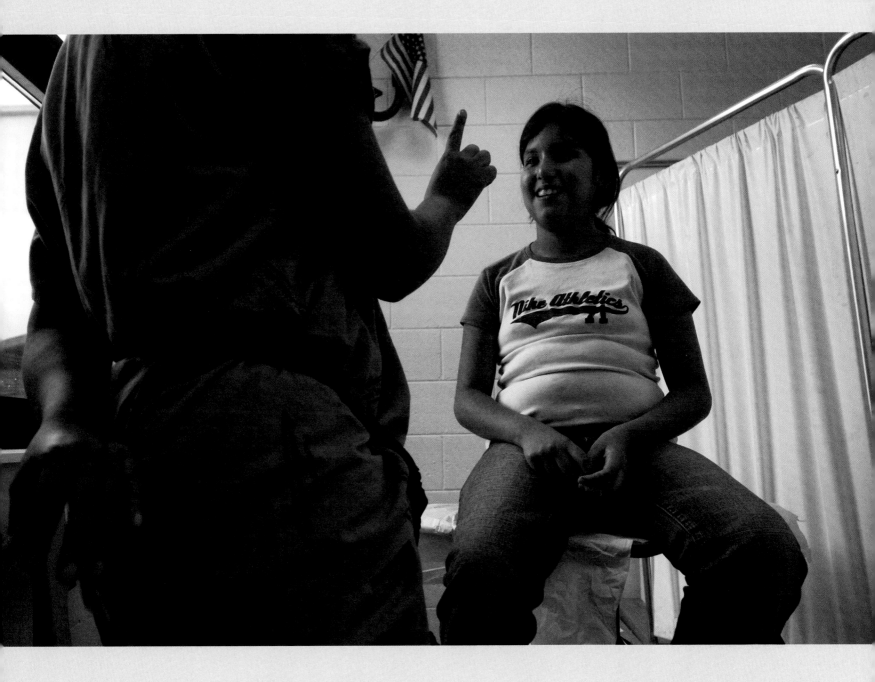

from their backbreaking labor. The volunteers get help with their work from the Ellenton Clinic in Moultrie and from area businesses, who donate supplies to the project and "goodie bags" to migrant families.

For Emory students, participation in the program reflects the nursing school's commitment to "integrate the values of service and responsibility with the nursing curriculum."

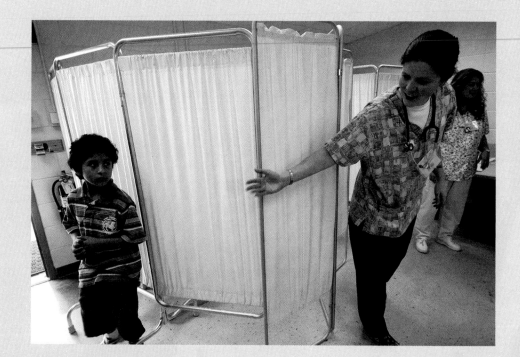

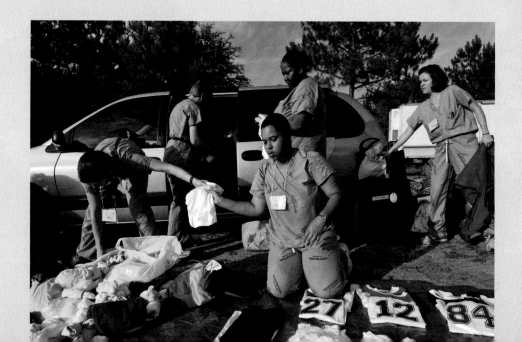

At a local school, volunteers provide basic health care to sometimes reluctant patients (top left). More enthusiastic, men (below) gather to sign up for free check-ups. Bottom left: Student nurses neatly arrange T-shirts and other used clothes, available for the taking.

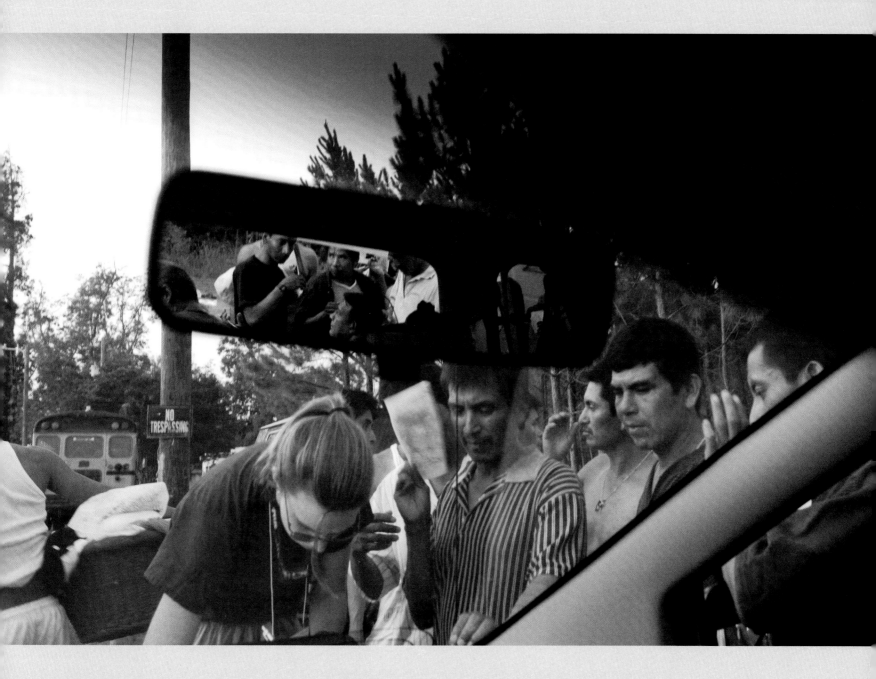

Nurses are pragmatists, problem solvers, improvisers, using the resources at hand to do what needs to be done. Sometimes they save lives by simply raising their voices. "I'm Bobbi Campbell," a registered nurse in San Francisco declared publicly in 1982, "and I have 'gay cancer.'" Campbell, 29 years old, was the sixteenth person in San Francisco diagnosed with Kaposi's sarcoma, a hitherto rare form of skin cancer that was spreading with terrible speed among gay men. More than a year would pass before the new disease was dubbed AIDS. During that time, so many young men were falling ill and dying that some hospital wards in the city looked like part of a war zone. Bobbi Campbell dedicated himself to warning the gay community in a series of articles written for a small newspaper called the *Sentinel.* He talked the local pharmacy into displaying a poster showing Kaposi's lesions so people would know how to recognize them. He used his experience as a nurse to advocate for the growing number of people with the new and terrifying disease. A statement he helped draft at the Second National AIDS Forum in 1983 declared: "We condemn attempts to label us as 'victims,' a term which implies defeat, and we are only occasionally 'patients,' a term which implies passivity, helplessness, and dependence upon the care of others. We are 'People With AIDS.'"

When nothing else worked, he used humor to get attention, christening himself Sister Florence Nightmare.

Two years after his diagnosis, Campbell died of complications from AIDS. In that brief time, his heroic efforts to alert the gay community to the danger in their midst saved uncounted lives. His torch is carried today by thousands of nurses working in parts of the world where the

Nurses are pragmatists, problem solvers, improvisers, using the resources at hand to do what needs to be done.

epidemic still rages—nurses like Cherry Matimuna in Kabwe, Zambia, who adopted her niece's and nephew's four children after their parents died of AIDS and then went on to help care for more than 60 other children orphaned by the disease. Attending the 16th International AIDS Conference in 2006 to crusade for more access to antiviral treatments and renewed efforts to stem the epidemic, she said, "We're fighting to create another strong generation."

SLOWLY BUT SURELY, THE VOICE OF NURSING HAS GAINED STRENGTH AND resolve, both collectively and through the work of individual pioneers. More than a century ago, the International Council of Nurses was formed to promote the development of the profession around the world. One of its most recent accomplishments was the creation of an international disaster response network, ready at a moment's notice to respond to health crises or disasters wherever they strike.

Meanwhile, nurses are beginning to be represented in the top ranks of the World Health Organization (WHO) and in governmental and non-governmental health organizations around the world. They are serving in roles that are exclusively held by nurses and, more recently, in roles that traditionally had been the exclusive domain of physicians. Nurses are now counted in the ranks of ministers of health and other key policy positions in both the developed and developing world, where they speak out for policies that create safe and supportive environments to provide nurses with the respect and resources they need to do their best work.

The voice of nursing is also being heard in scientific circles, where nurses are advancing care through research extending from the bench

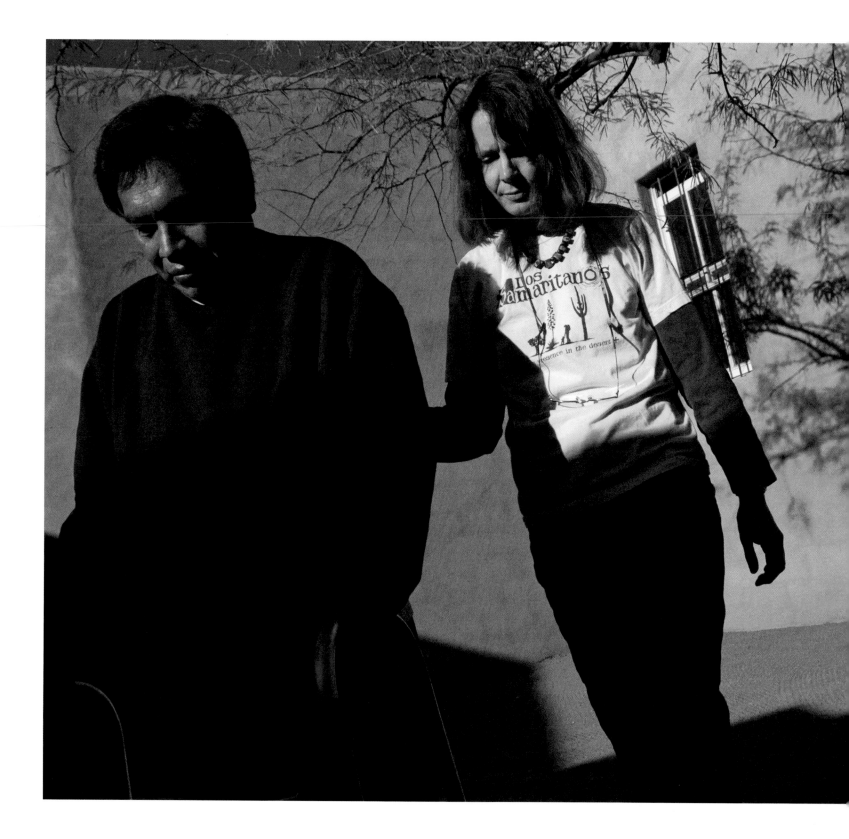

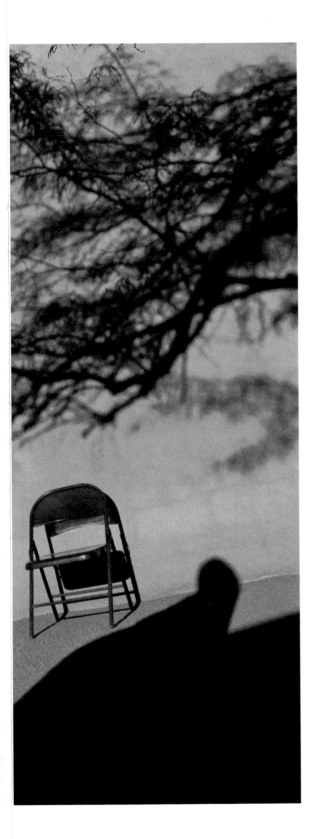

Their name—Samaritans—says it all. All volunteers, like this school nurse, they roam the Sonoran Desert of Arizona, looking for undocumented immigrants who are lost or injured in the desert. The Samaritans offer them food, water, and emergency medical care, but aren't allowed by law to offer transportation. This man lost part of his foot while jumping from a train and has just gotten the medical attention he needs to heal.

to the bedside. Their work has helped win new respect for nursing's contribution to patient health and safety and has shed light on ways to improve the quality of bedside care.

Behind these powerful voices are millions of practicing nurses who speak as nurses always have, not through words but actions—nurses like Sarah Roberts, who worked as a medical-surgical nurse in Tucson, Arizona, for 18 years and then became a school nurse so that she could be an advocate for families in an increasingly complex health care system. On her days off, she's part of the Samaritan Patrol—nurses and other volunteers who provide food, water, and emergency medical care to people crossing the border. The people she serves are known by some as illegal aliens. To Roberts, they are simply human beings desperate enough for a better life that they risk death in the killing heat of the Arizona desert—people who deserve compassion and help.

"When I first thought of nursing, I wanted a career and skills I could use to help people in a really basic way, at a time when they were most vulnerable," explained Roberts. "To be a healing presence in people's lives. That's the gift of nursing. And it's a gift that you get to give and receive."

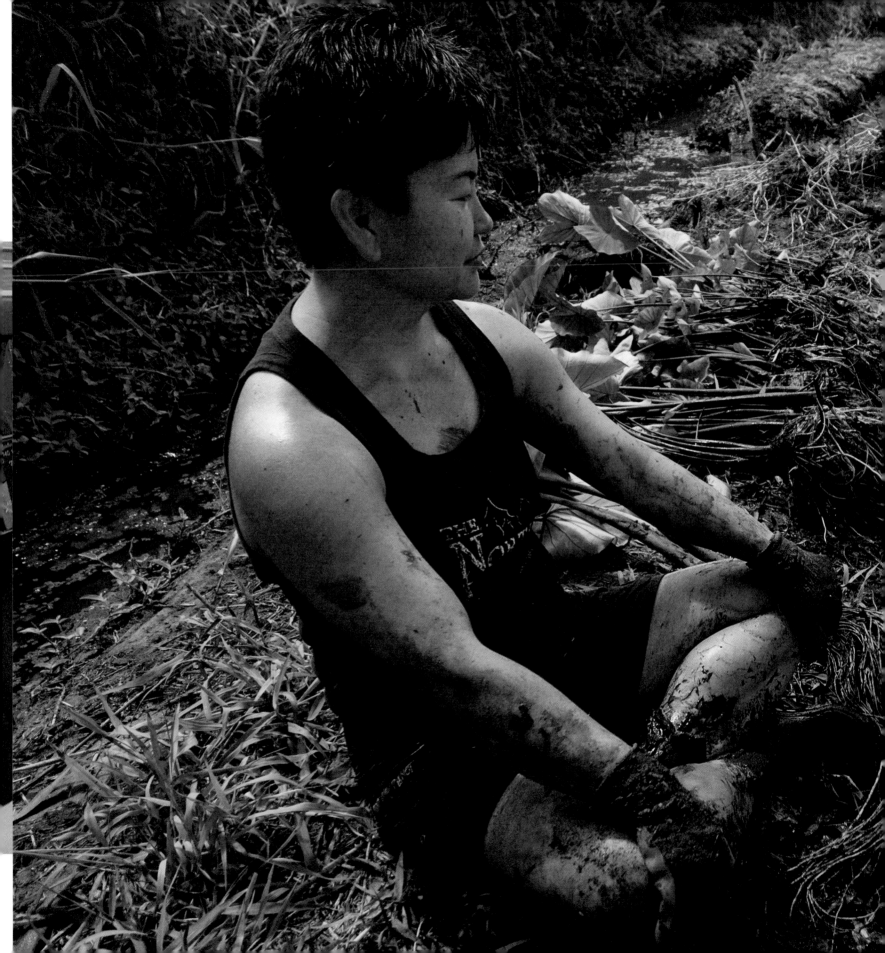

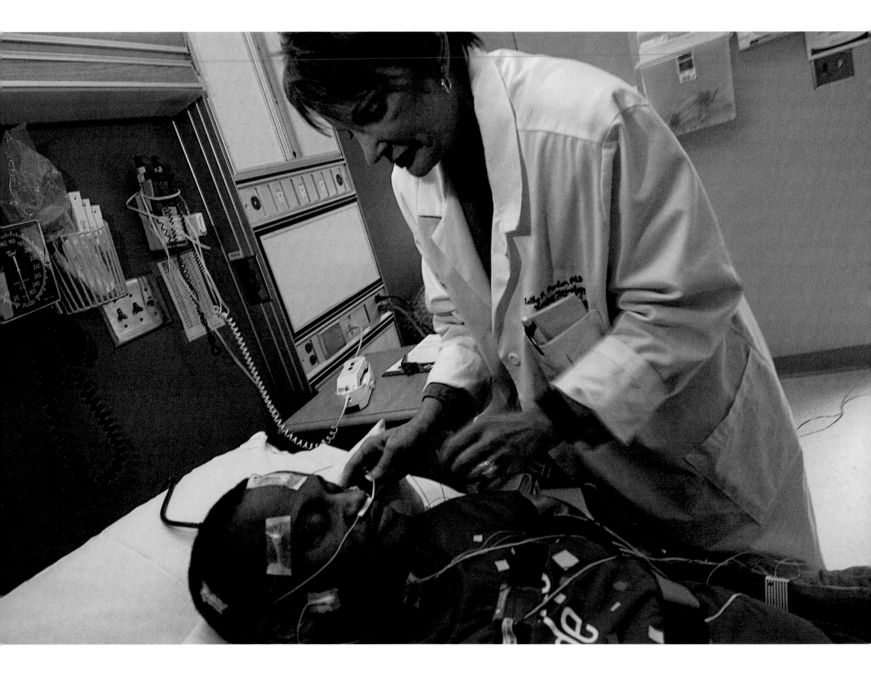

TWO

ADVANCING THE PROFESSION

"A good Nurse," Florence Nightingale wrote in an 1878 letter to her students, "will test her Nursing & learn something to the last day of her Nursing life." Many nurses have been inspired by Nightingale's example, advancing the profession in ways that would have gratified and delighted her. Certainly she would have been enthralled to watch a critical-care nurse in a pediatric intensive care unit, monitoring lifesaving equipment unimaginable a century ago. She would have been overjoyed to discover a Reno, Nevada, clinic run entirely by nurses, who diagnose and treat poor and disadvantaged people. No doubt she would have understood exactly the sense of a higher calling that leads a young nurse from a privileged family to risk her life treating victims of war in the Congo. And she would have smiled with undisguised pleasure to see critical-care nurses at Emory University Hospital in Atlanta, Georgia, playing a key role in designing a new state-of-the-art neurology intensive care unit to treat patients who have suffered severe brain injury, strokes, and aneurysms.

Nightingale would have marveled at all that nursing has become in the 21st century—a profession that combines advanced practice, research, a long history, and a rich vein of philosophy.

Sleep disorders, both vexing and debilitating, are a growing problem for many. At a clinic run by Emory University's pioneering sleep medicine program, Kathy Parker, a nurse scientist, monitors the brain waves of people hoping for treatment and answers. Her research is helping find those answers.

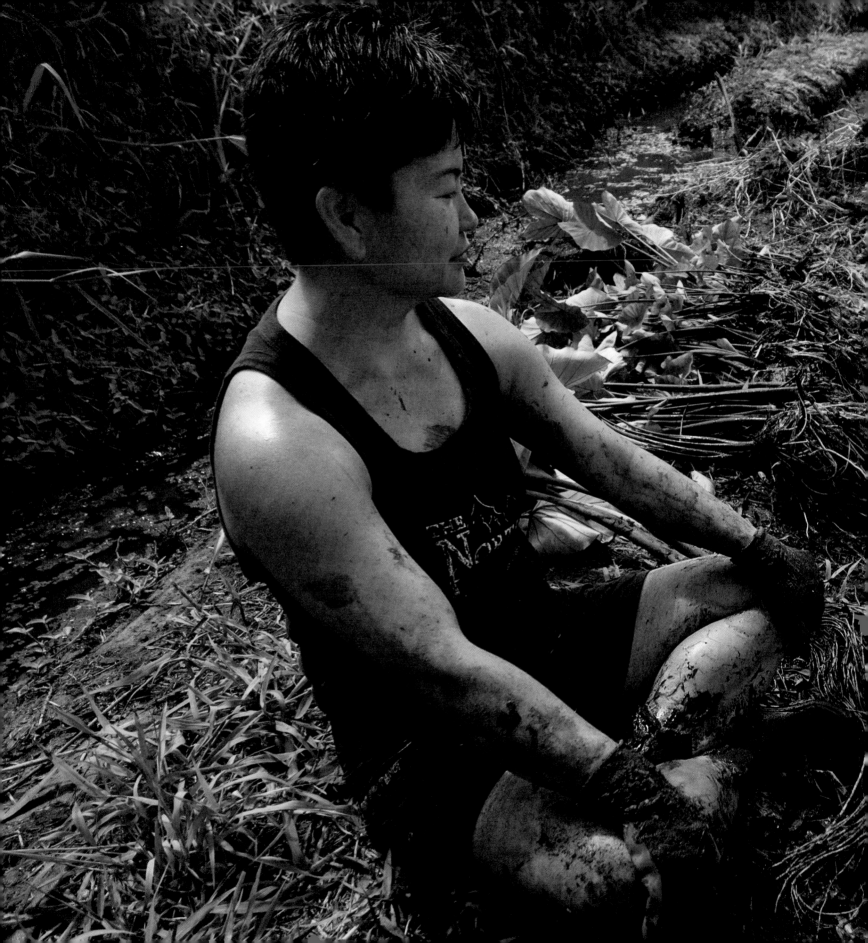

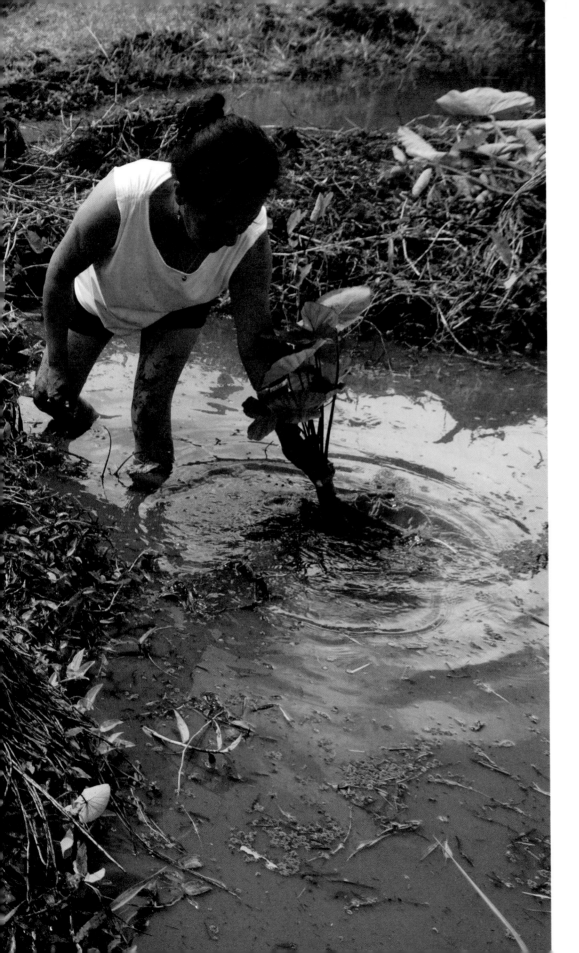

As a public health nurse on Oahu, Joan Takamori (left) knows that the more she understands the Hawaiian culture, the better able she'll be to treat the health problems of native Hawaiians. So she and her nursing students spend a day in the taro fields, learning from Hawaiians themselves what this sacred plant, "brother of mankind," means to the culture.

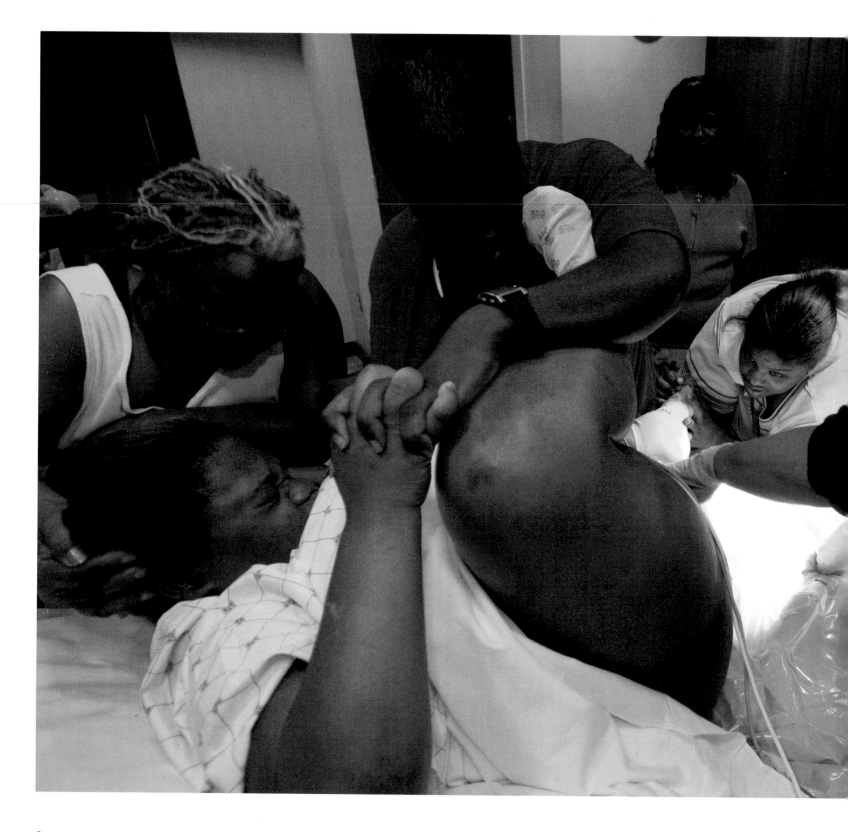

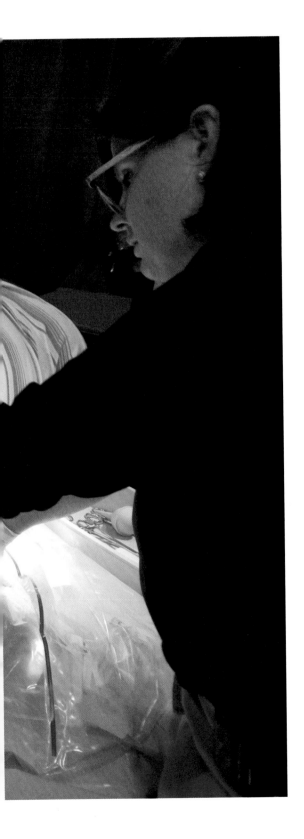

The remarkable progress of nursing parallels and reflects the rapid advances that have transformed medicine itself. During Nightingale's life, precious few effective medicines existed. Medical care was based largely on anecdotal evidence. By far the most powerful technology for saving lives was basic sanitation. The tools available were often as simple as soap, a bandage, and a soothing word, as Louisa May Alcott's poignant description of her nursing work after the battle at Fredericksburg, Virginia, in 1863 attests: "I had managed to sort out the patients in such a way that I had what I called 'my duty room', 'my pleasure room', and 'my pathetic room' . . . . One I visited armed with a dressing tray full of rollers, plasters, and pins; another, with books, flowers, games, and gossip; a third, with teapots, lullabies, consolation, and sometimes a shroud."

In the 80 years following the Civil War, the work and responsibilities of nursing underwent a revolution. In 1942, University of Rochester nursing researcher Claire Dennison scrupulously documented the procedures and treatments performed by nurses over a 24-hour period at a large teaching hospital. Among 473 patients, 109 had to have blood pressure checked, some every 15 minutes. Sixty had to be given fluids or blood transfusions. Seven were on oxygen therapy. The nurses applied 230 dressings and administered 1,500 medications by mouth or

Bringing new life into the world, nurse midwife Laura Holbrook, far right, acts as primary care giver at Family Health and Birth Center in Washington, D.C., while Doris Denman—a traditional doula, or coach— sits at the mother's head encouraging her.

injection. In the midst of all these responsibilities, Dennison wrote, "it was understood that the nurses would know how to administer any drug—and pick up any error in writing the order."

Today, some 60 years after Dennison's landmark analysis, the practice of nursing has been transformed once again. On general medical wards and in extended-care facilities, nurses routinely supervise for the treatment of patients who are on six or seven different medications, each with its own complex dosing schedule and potential interactions. Diabetic patients may need frequent treatment for diabetic ulcers. Bedridden patients have to be watched for pressure ulcers and early signs of pneumonia. In a typical critical-care unit, nurses monitor not only heart rate, respiratory rate, and temperature but also hemodynamic pressure, oxygen saturation, carbon dioxide levels, and complex heart rhythms. They have to be trained in the use of defibrillators, infusion pumps, mechanical ventilators, and a host of other technologies.

One response to the growing complexity of medical care has been the emergence of specialties in advanced-practice nursing, which allows nurses to gain additional expertise and responsibility by combining basic nursing education with graduate-level training in particular areas. Clinical nurse specialists can focus on any of a wide range of fields, including cardiology, oncology, emergency medicine, neonatology, pediatrics, and mental health. Some nurses have pursued advanced degrees in public health; others in health care administration. Specialization in nursing has given rise to whole new fields as well, such as psychiatric nursing, forensic nursing, informatics nursing, and genomics nursing.

The growth of advanced-practice nursing has been driven by more

Around the
world, nursing
is taking on
new roles and
responsibilities
in order to meet
the profession's
enduring commit-
ment to providing
care for everyone
in need.

than just advances in medicine, however. An equally powerful push comes from a very different direction: growing inequities in access to health care around the world. In the U.S., for example, nurse practitioners, who receive additional graduate-level education that enables them to diagnose diseases and prescribe medication, are increasingly filling the gap left by the declining number of family physicians. Their ranks expanded significantly starting in the 1990s, especially in neglected communities—in rural clinics or homeless shelters, for instance, where physician care is often not available. They also play important roles in many nonprofit health-related organizations that work in developing countries.

Many nurses have specialized in the use of anesthesia simply because physician anesthesiologists weren't available in underserved communities. More than 75 years ago, the American Association of Nurse Anesthetists came into being to represent the new specialty. Today, nurse anesthetists administer approximately 27 million anesthetics a year in the U.S. alone. In almost all rural hospitals, they are the sole anesthesia providers. They have also played a critical role during wartime.

Certified nurse midwives also arose to address gaps in health care, both in remote areas of the country and in impoverished urban communities. Following in the footsteps of Lillian Wald, who brought health care to the squalid tenements of New York in the early 20th century, a young nurse and midwife named Ruth Lubic founded the first state-licensed birthing center in New York City's Upper East Side in 1975. In 1988, she opened another in the South Bronx, one of the city's poorest neighborhoods. Both centers ignited a furor of protest from physicians, who insisted that midwives couldn't deliver babies safely. Lubic had to fight to keep the centers open.

She prevailed. In 2000, after winning a prestigious MacArthur Foundation Fellows Program "genius grant," Lubic opened a second facility in an abandoned grocery store building in Washington, D.C., and called it the DC Developing Families Center, a name that speaks not only to Lubic's personal mission but to one of nursing's age-old values. "Every time a baby is born," Lubic said when the center opened, "hope comes back and strengthens families."

Around the world, nursing is taking on new roles and responsibilities in order to meet the profession's enduring commitment to providing care for everyone in need. The island nation of Cuba provides a powerful example. During the 1959 revolution, half of all physicians and many nurses left the island, creating an acute medical crisis. To achieve the government's ambitious goal of universal health care, midwives trained to become nurse's aides. Aides went on to become nurses. Nurses took on advanced-practice specialties. Today, Cuba serves as a model for delivering health care with limited resources. Its success story is being replicated in other developing nations, where nurses have taken the lead in building community health capacity by training a network of local caregivers. In Bangladesh, for example, village health care workers, trained by nurses to provide basic care, have vastly extended medicine's reach into the most isolated rural areas, reducing risks of diarrheal disease and other chronic and life-threatening conditions. In parts of sub-Saharan Africa, nurses are expanding their reach by teaching village health workers how to administer and monitor lifesaving HIV/AIDS drugs.

The rise of advanced-practice nursing has been accompanied by another welcome change: a closer partnership between physicians and

Nurse midwife Lisa Uncles examines a newborn at the Family Health and Birth Center, founded by nurse midwife Ruth Lubic in 2000. Since time immemorial women have helped other women give birth, but in the 20th century, the functions of midwifes were often usurped by doctors. Today, nurse midwives are meeting the needs of women in a variety of situations. And centers—frequently, like this one, serving the urban poor—have made great strides in improving infant and maternal health.

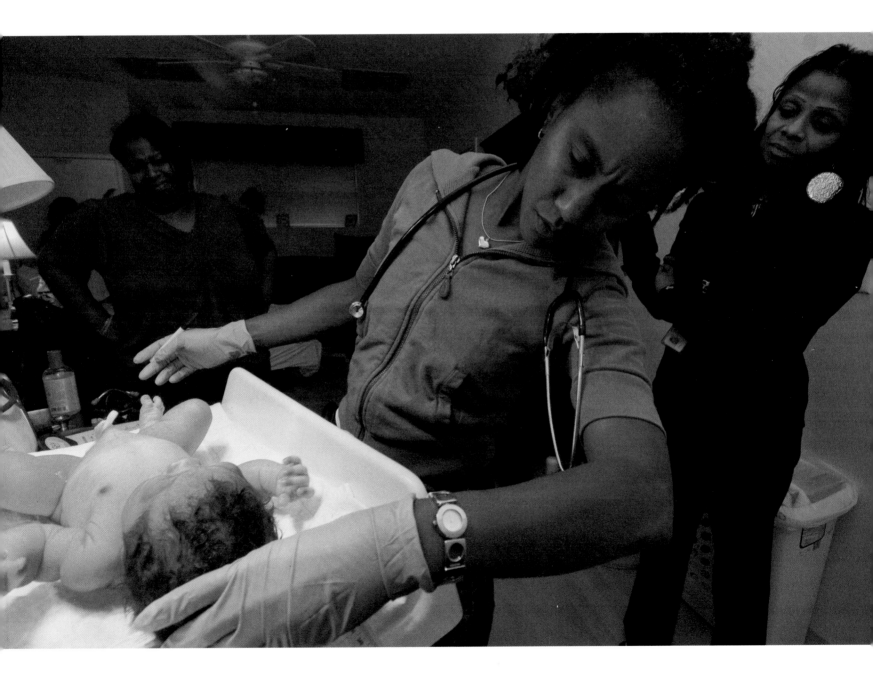

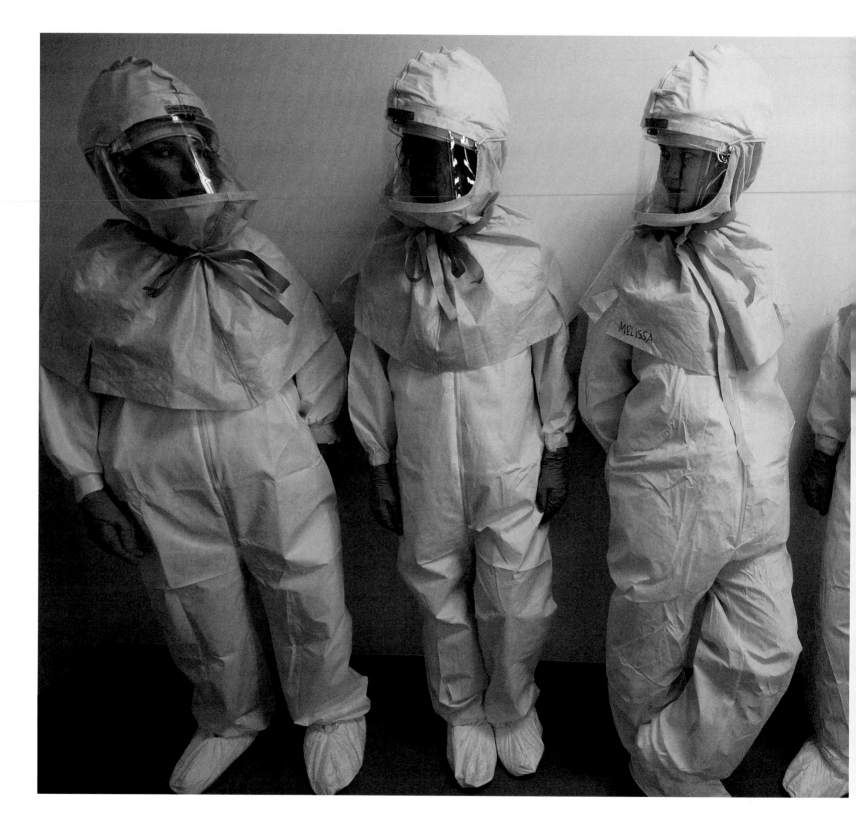

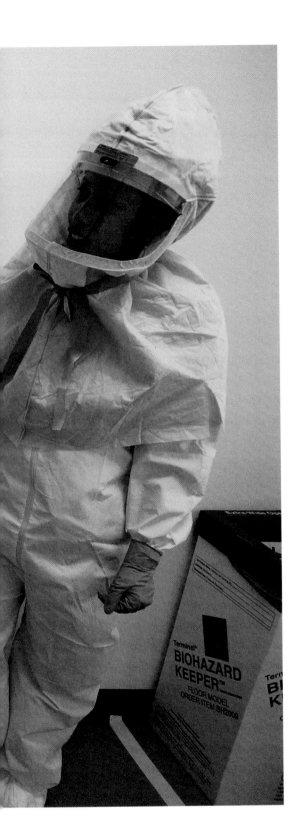

Heading off potential new challenges, nursing students now learn to function in awkward "hazmat" suits. Should there be a medical emergency in one of the many biohazard labs now proliferating across the U.S., nurses will be among the first responders.

nurses. Although the two disciplines have always worked together, the relationship hasn't always been easy. Nurses frequently bridle at a lack of respect for their work. Physicians have often resisted the attempts of nurses to take on more responsibility, especially where it encroaches on the traditional areas of a doctor's expertise. These tensions haven't been banished. But many nurses say there is a healthy and growing spirit of cooperation and mutual respect. In more and more hospitals and health care facilities, physicians and nurses work as a team to shape treatment and ensure patient safety. In the developing world, a closer alliance between doctors and nurses is making it possible to deliver health care despite very limited resources. Here, again, Cuba provides a powerful example. On the island, primary care is typically delivered by doctor-nurse teams, often living in the communities they serve. By making home visits together, physicians and nurses enable many patients who would otherwise have to be hospitalized to remain with their families, preserving their quality of life and at the same time saving money. The team approach encourages close communication and a consistent treatment plan while also allowing nurses to extend their own expertise and responsibilities. The model has led to remarkably high immunization rates and early prevention or control of chronic and communicable diseases—in short, to healthier communities.

"Hospitals," the physician and essayist Lewis Thomas wrote, "are held together, glued together, enabled to function . . . by the nurses." Nurses have always served as the bridge between doctors and patients, carrying out orders as well as observing patients and alerting physicians to signs of trouble. Today that role is more complex and demanding than ever before.

Hospitalized patients are often seen by two or more physician specialists. Their care typically includes a variety of medications and the use of multiple technologies, from monitoring equipment to periodic tests. Information has to be conveyed among physicians, patients, and family members, frequently during times of wrenching emotional distress. Nurses need to possess not only technical expertise but also the traditional "people" skills of intuition, communication, and negotiation. Nurses, in other words, aren't so much the glue as they are the gaskets that allow all the complex parts of the medical machinery to function together smoothly.

THE METAPHOR OF MODERN HEALTH CARE AS A MACHINE IS ALMOST TOO APT. The practice of medicine has become so dependent on advanced technologies that many patients complain about feeling lost and depersonalized once they enter the medical system. When the system itself is ailing, as it is in many countries—when patients have to battle insurance companies, suffer long waiting periods for treatment, or live in fear of ruinous medical bills—the situation can be fraught with anger and anxiety. And so nurses are increasingly being called on to preserve the human face of health care, to stand as a buffer between patients and the medical system itself, to protect and defend patients' essential human dignity. Nurses listen, explain, console, and sometimes sooth a patient's anxieties with nothing more than a reassuring word or a gentle touch. They are there when no one else is, late in the night, early in the morning, not only for patients but for their families as well.

"Nurses are the heart and soul of health care," said Hermi Hewitt, who directs the University of the West Indies *Continued on page 100*

"You're sick, we're quick." That's the idea behind retail health clinics like this "MinuteClinic" in Rockville, Maryland. Offered by the CVS drugstore chain, MinuteClinics have nurse practitioners on hand to treat walk-in patients with common complaints—colds, flu, infections—and to give inoculations, take blood pressure, and write some prescriptions. Such accessible, affordable care could prevent illnesses and the complications that arise from untreated or undiagnosed health problems.

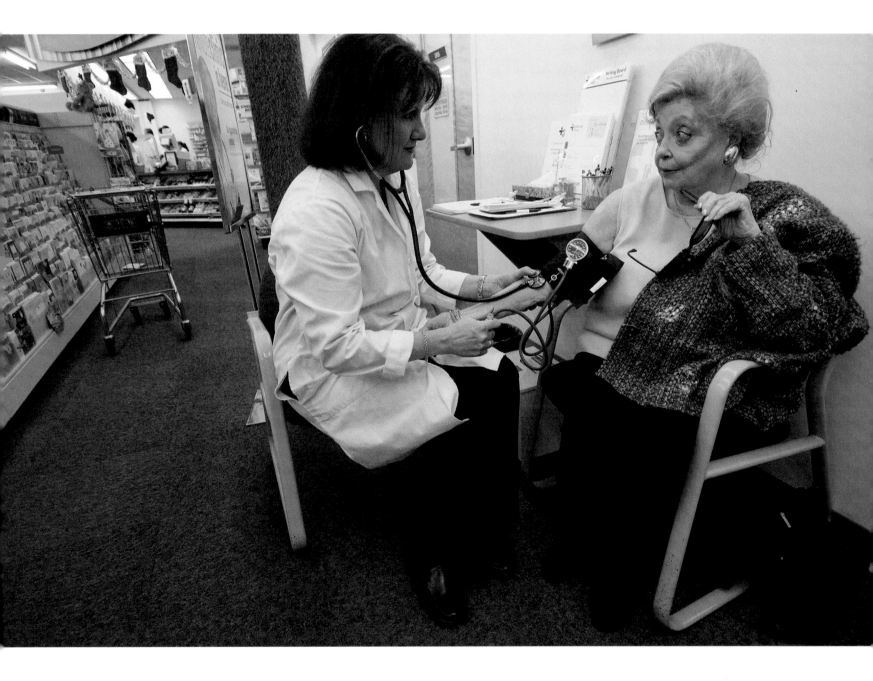

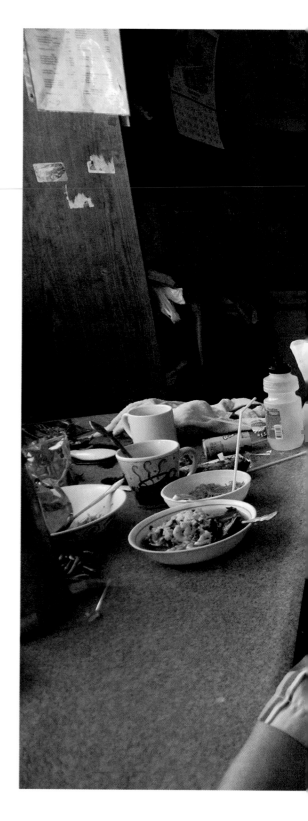

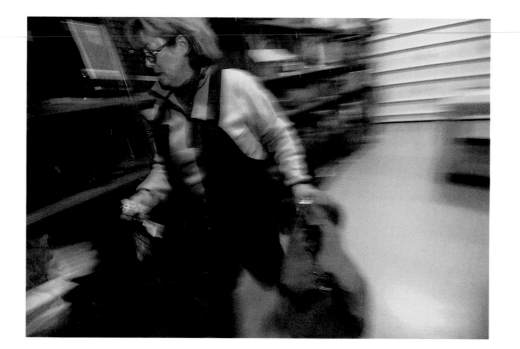

Nurse on the go, Mary Berliner has to pack in everything she needs to visit the clinics she maintains, scattered across a remote area of south-western Alaska. Among her clients is the elderly man at right, whose family asked Mary to make a home visit. Public health nurses serve as primary health providers in much of Alaska, stationing themselves in bare-bones clinics in native Alaskan communities for a week at a time, living out of a backpack, and spreading a sleeping bag at night. Most nurses caring for these isolated communities last only a couple of years, but Mary has been on the job for more than a decade now.

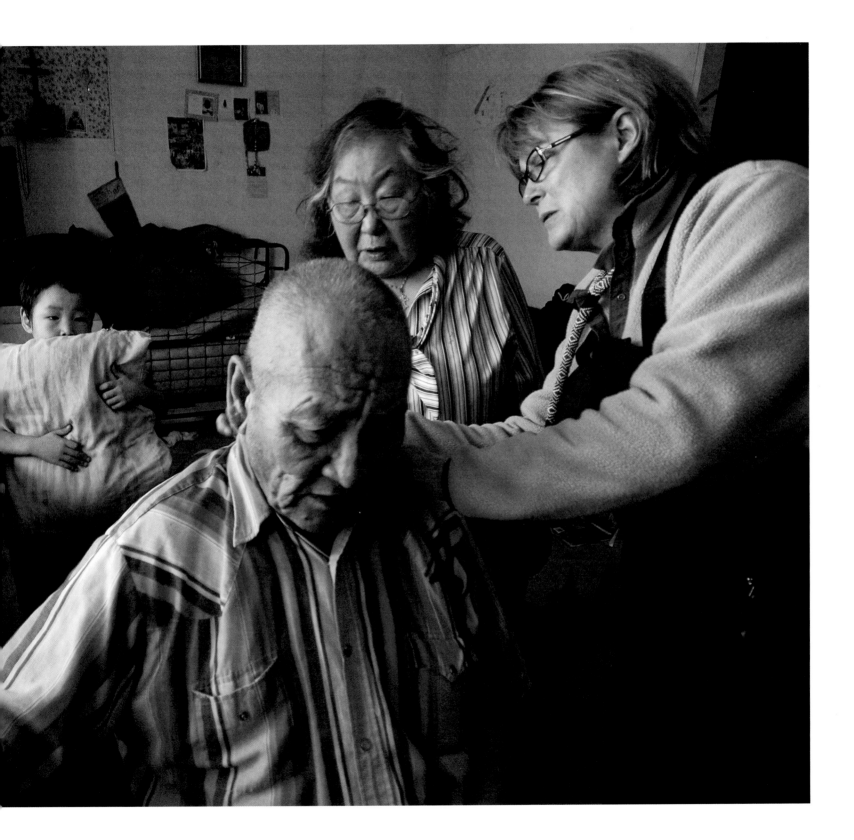

Frozen rivers become roads during the long dark Alaska winter. Public health nurses travel these ice roads to visit communities close to their home base. For more distant communities, nurses rely on the small planes that act as a connective lifeline throughout Alaska.

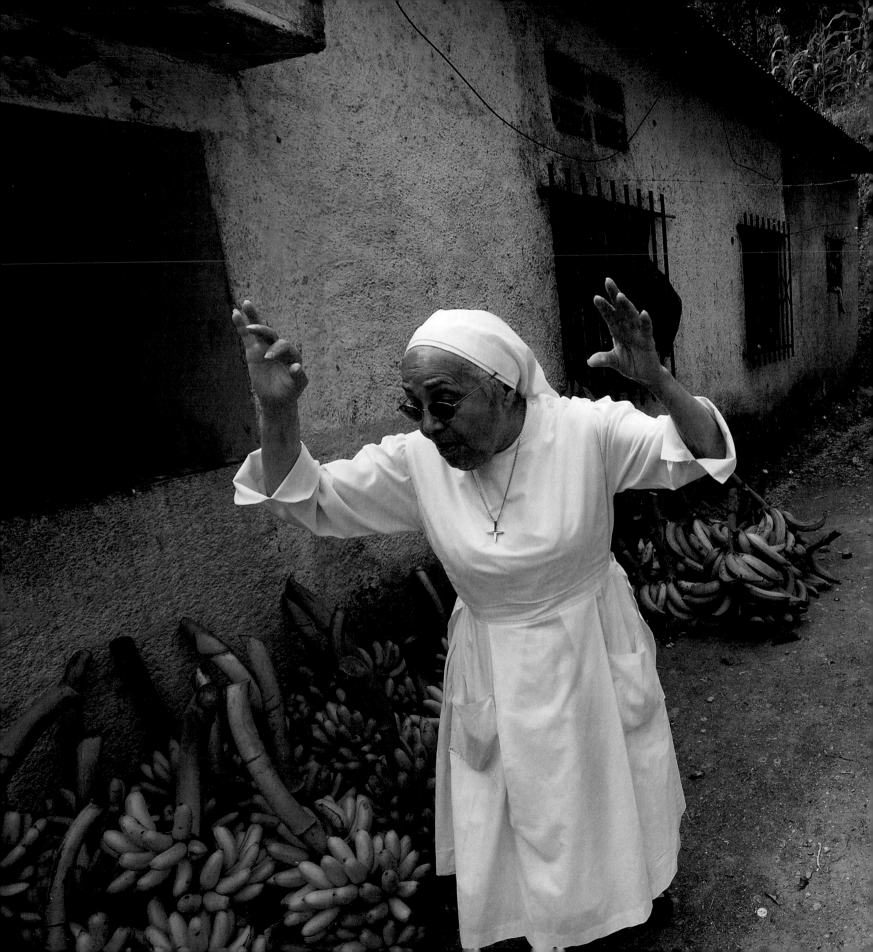

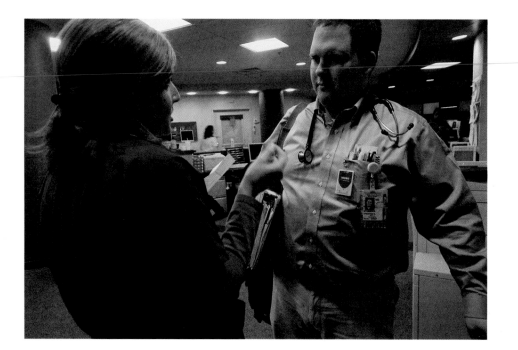

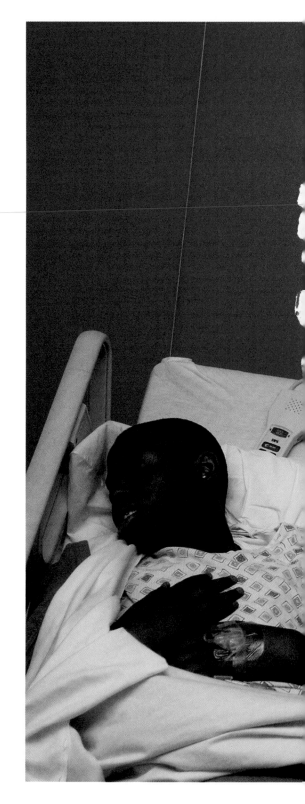

Tough but rewarding work: Erin Connelly (above and right) knows only
too well the stress of nursing in a pediatric cancer ward. Before becoming a nurse, Erin briefly pursued a career in banking, but the death of
one of her closest friends led her to change careers. Her work, she says,
keeps her life in perspective. "I really am so privileged— I recognize what a
responsibility I have to other human beings."

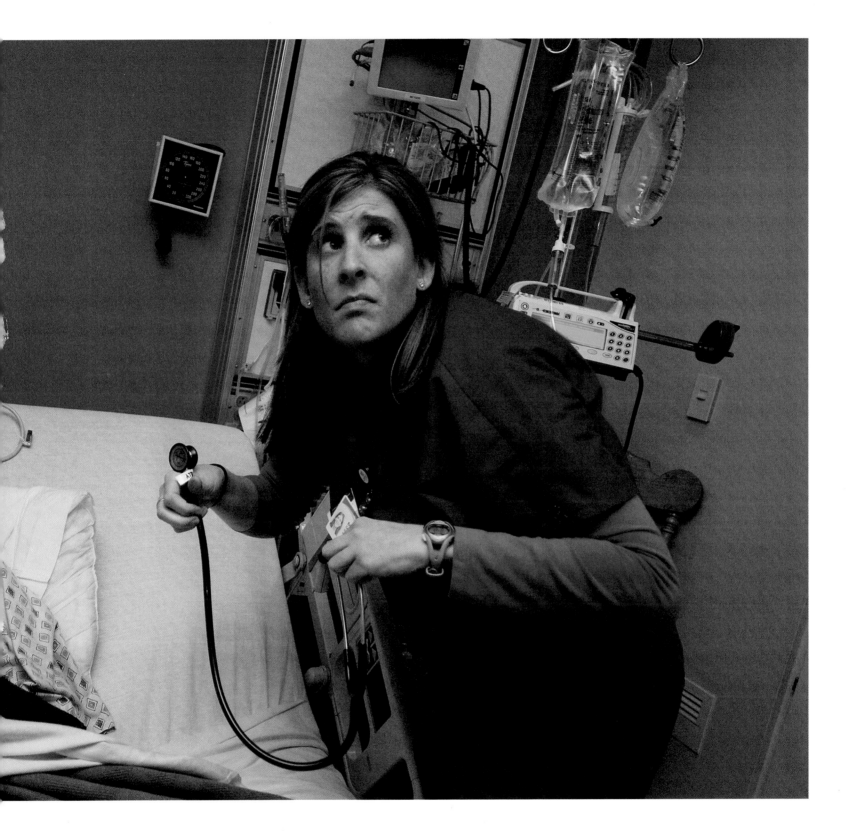

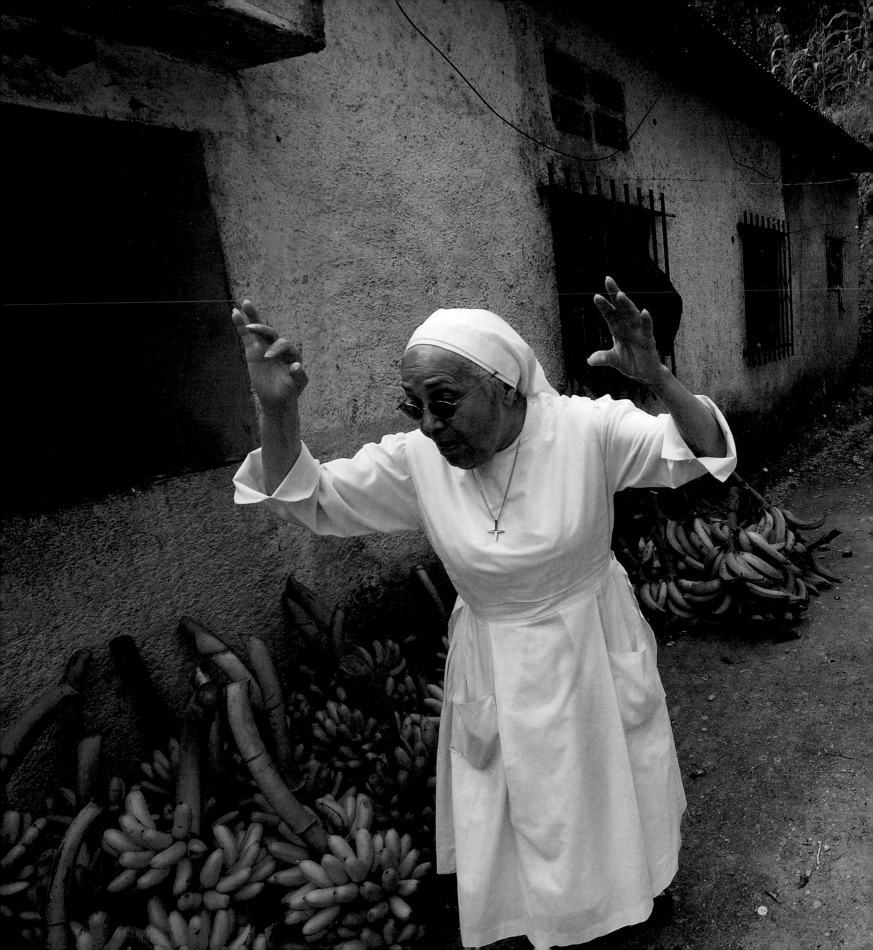

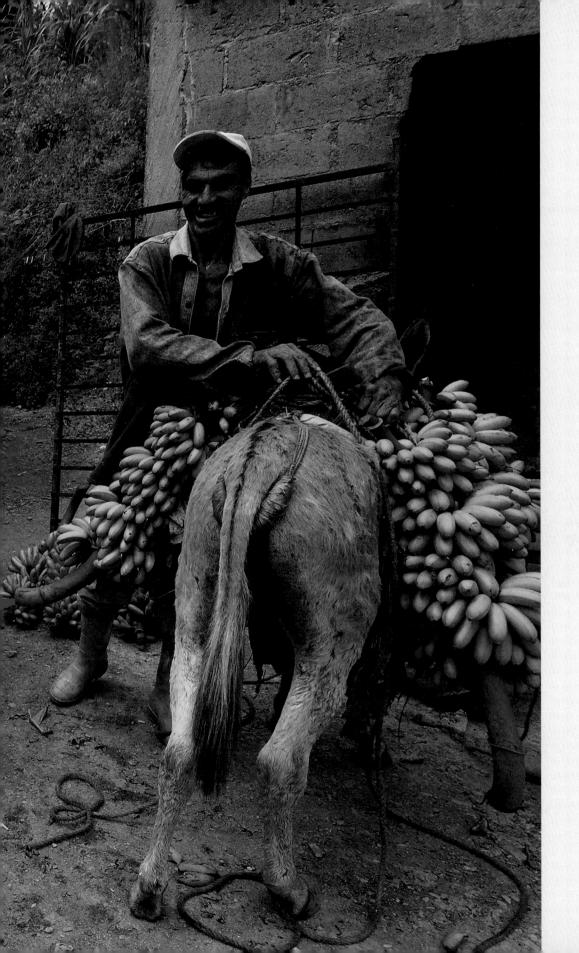

A SISTER'S PASSION

Eighty-year-old Sister Isolena came to nursing later in life. But she's more than made up for lost time. From her convent base in Caracas, the nurse and nun now serves a wide community scattered across northeastern Venezuela. Both a field nurse and a researcher, she visits those who need care and works on ways to combat parasitic diseases, many of them related to bad water and the marshy conditions here.

Life hasn't changed much for the Warao of the Orinoco

Throwing up her hands, Sister Isolena finally gives in to a local banana seller, who, out of respect, refuses to accept payment from her for his wares.

Delta since the Spanish first
sailed up the river in 1494.
Most still live in open-sided,
thatched-roof huts on stilts
built over the river. They travel
the threaded waterways
of their world by dugout
canoe, and they're shadowed
by malnourishment, disease,
and early death. With logging
and oil interests now exploit-
ing their lands, many are
migrating to cities, where poverty continues to plague them.

Sister Isolena travels the
isolated, often dangerous
world of the Warao, visiting
homes and the few clinics
that operate here. Beyond just
medicine, she represents a
caring face from a land outside
the Warao realm.

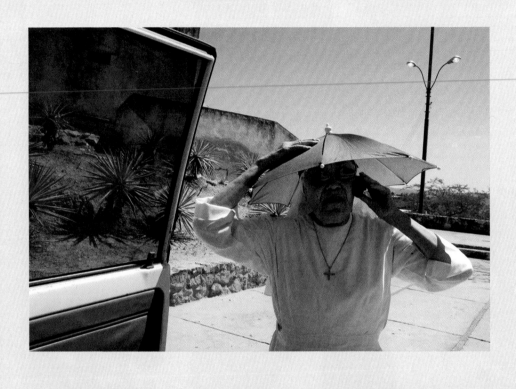

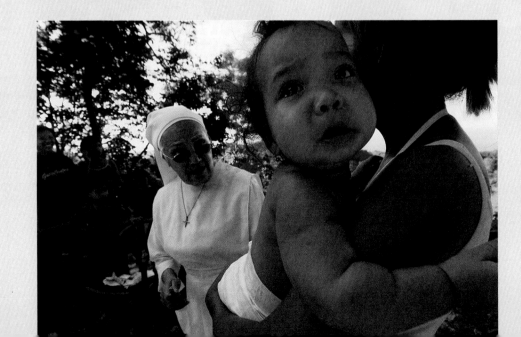

For the Warao of the Orinoco Delta, the river provides water for every-thing—drinking, brushing teeth, cooking, washing—and that makes it a perfect vector for disease. Too busy treating these people to worry about sun or rain, Sister Isolena wears an umbrella hat (left) that can handle all weathers. When she arrives in an area, word quickly spreads, often resulting in a spontaneous roadside clinic (bottom).

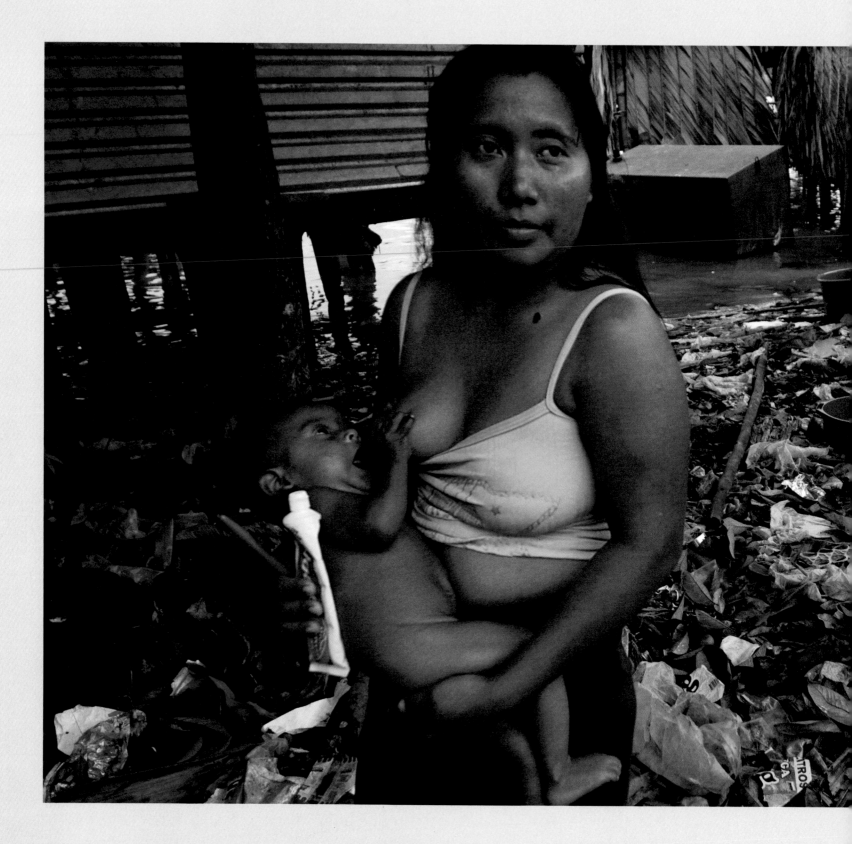

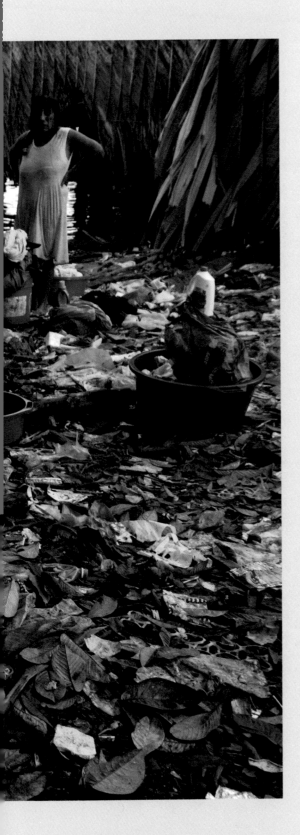

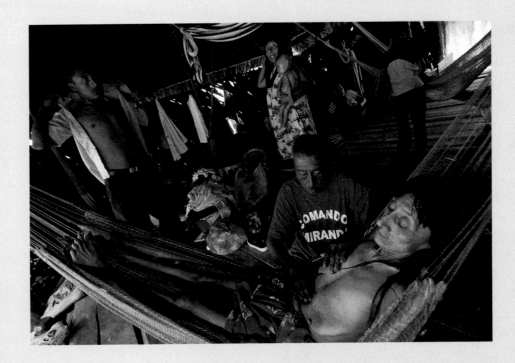

Tide's out, and the trash-laden shores of the Orinoco are exposed (left). Most Warao women have a number of babies, but infant mortality is high and female life expectancy low. Nurses in the area have to combat not only a host of illnesses but traditional beliefs as well. The woman above has sought treatment from a local shaman, to rid her of the "spells" causing her illness.

School of Nursing, Mona campus, in Kingston, Jamaica. "They create the bubble of comfort and support that surrounds patients when they are at their most vulnerable." That role extends far beyond the hospital. Increasingly, home health care nurses serve as the bridge between hospital care and home care once patients are discharged, especially as lengths of hospital stays are being reduced to save health care dollars. "It's really nurses who help patients make the transition from hospital to home. They're the ones who preserve continuity of care," explained Hewitt, who is currently working to create a stronger structure for home health care in the Caribbean.

Nurses have always been part teacher, part guide, making sure that patients understand their diagnoses and treatments. Now they are taking on a related role, as well: that of helping patients decide the kind and level of care they want. "Traditionally, health care providers have told patients what the goal should be," says Susan Grant, who is Chief Nurse at Emory Healthcare in Atlanta. "But the outcome that patients and family want may be very different from what their provider wants, and more and more nurses can play a pivotal role in ensuring that the patient and family are involved in making those decisions." A patient and family might decide to forego further treatment for a terminal illness in order to spend their last days together at home, for example.

The nurse's role is likely to become even more challenging as medicine extends its ability to diagnose subtypes of diseases—each with its own characteristics—and as treatment regimens become more complex. With advances in genetic research making it possible to identify the inherited risk of such serious disorders as Huntington's disease, breast cancer, and amyotrophic lateral sclerosis (Lou Gehrig's disease) years

Nurse Hob Osterlund dons the wig, uniform, and comic persona of Ivy Push, RN, to administer a little of the laugh therapy she practices on patients at the Queen's Medical Center in Honolulu.

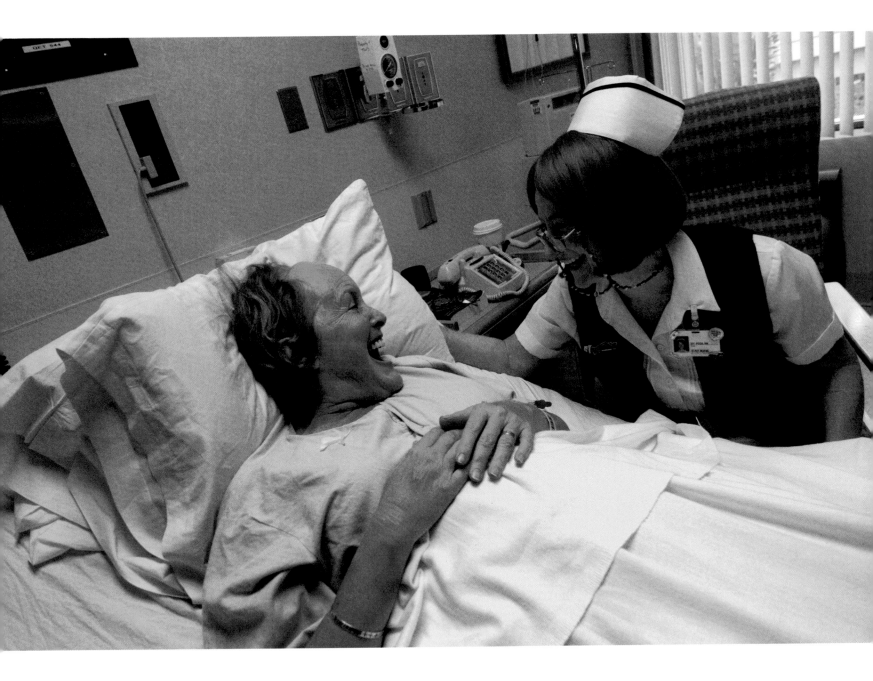

before they show up, the role of teacher and counselor will require ever greater sensitivity and compassion.

IN COUNTRIES WHERE WOMEN ARE FREE TO CHOOSE AMONG A GROWING RANGE of occupations, nurses are finding completely new and novel ways to use their training and expertise. Some have pursued business and management degrees in order to take on leading roles in running health care companies and organizations. Nurse attorneys combine RN degrees with legal degrees in order to specialize in health care law and policy. More and more nurses are becoming entrepreneurs in their own right, founding a wide range of nursing-related companies, from health publishing to medical equipment design. In the face of growing shortages of nurses in many hospitals, some enterprising nurses have launched staffing companies.

The new range of opportunities has transformed the professional lives of many nurses, often in ways they would never have imagined. As a student in the West African nation of the Ivory Coast, Maimouna Toure-Keita dreamed of being a nurse or midwife. Before she had the chance, however, she and her husband immigrated to Minnesota, where he took a job as a college professor. When their second child was born with severe birth defects, they spent long hours in hospitals. "The nurses who looked after my daughter were so caring that I began to think again about becoming a nurse," remembered Toure-Keita.

She did. First she served as a nurse's assistant in a nursing home. Then she went back to school to become a registered nurse. After working as an RN for almost 14 years, Toure-Keita returned to school to earn a BSN (Bachelor of Science in Nursing) and then became a nurse

More than mere pests, lice pose a real health problem. So these women, new immigrants to Hawaii from other Pacific islands, listen carefully as a public health nurse explains how to deal with the pesky parasites.

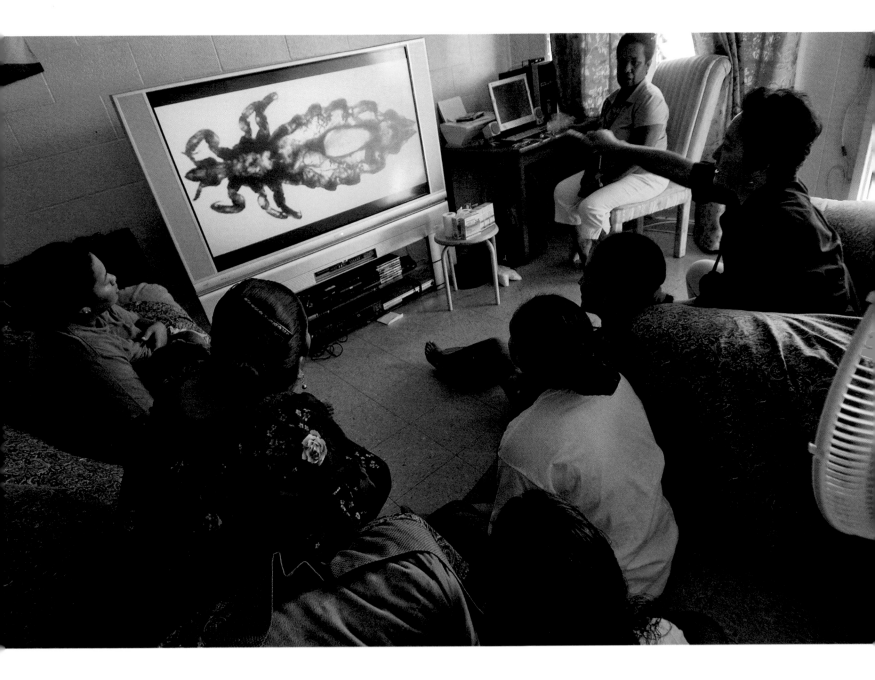

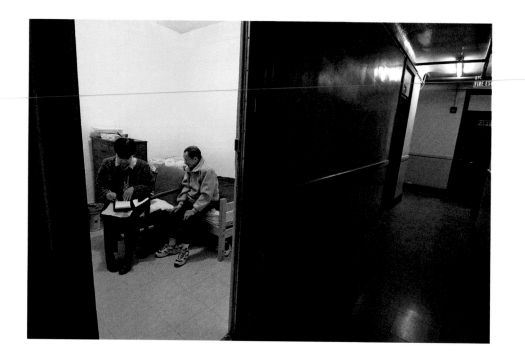

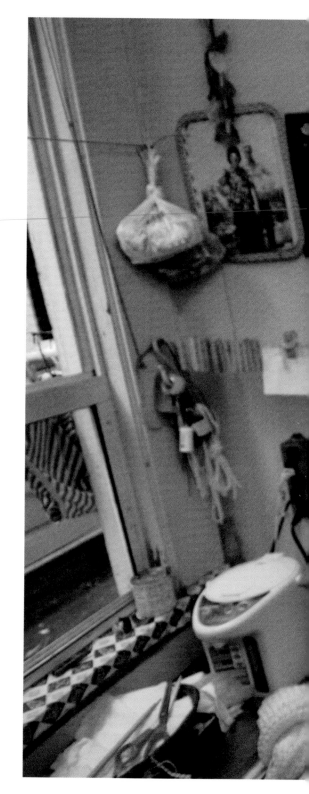

In San Francisco's Chinatown, the elderly can enjoy companionship and the freedom of living in their own small but adequate single-room apartments (right and above)—thanks to the groundbreaking services of On Lok. Founded here almost 40 years ago in response to an aging, multiethnic population, On Lok understands that cultural awareness is critical to good senior care, so its nurses and doctors are also ethnically diverse and able to speak the languages, literally and metaphorically, of its elderly participants.

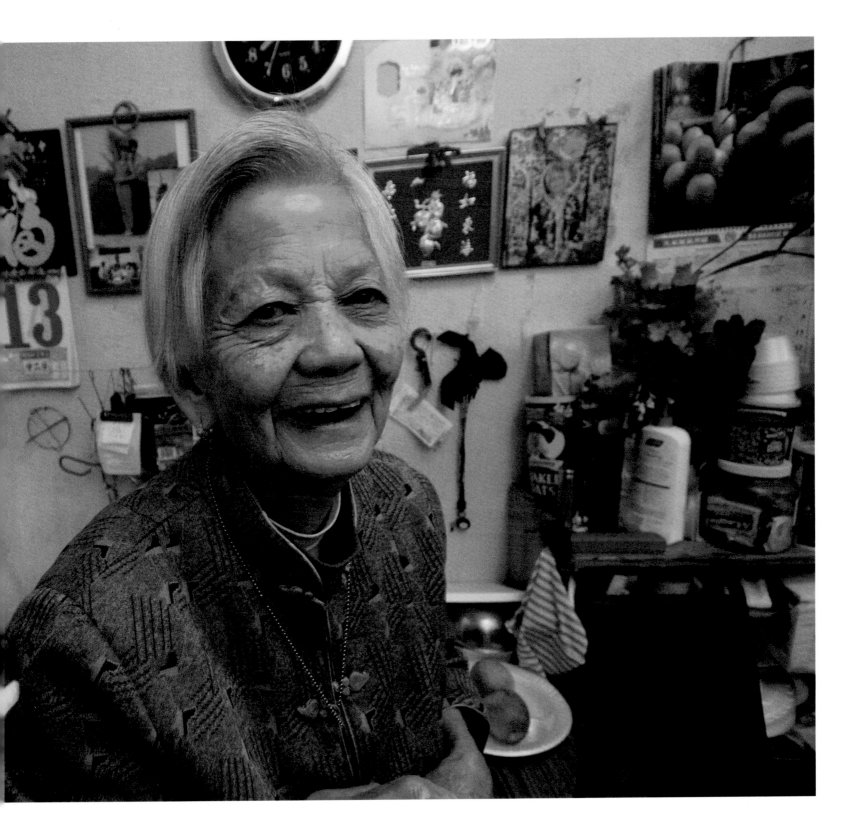

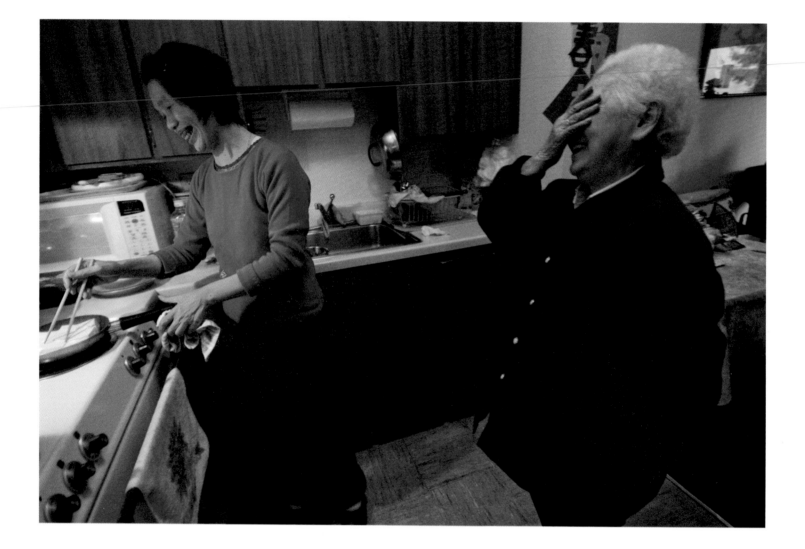

On Lok participants can opt for a wide variety of care, from home visits by aides who even prepare meals (left), to nursing care in the home, to days spent at a senior daycare center (below), where the generations often mix together. The On Lok concept has proved so successful that senior-care models based on it now operate in a number of U.S. states.

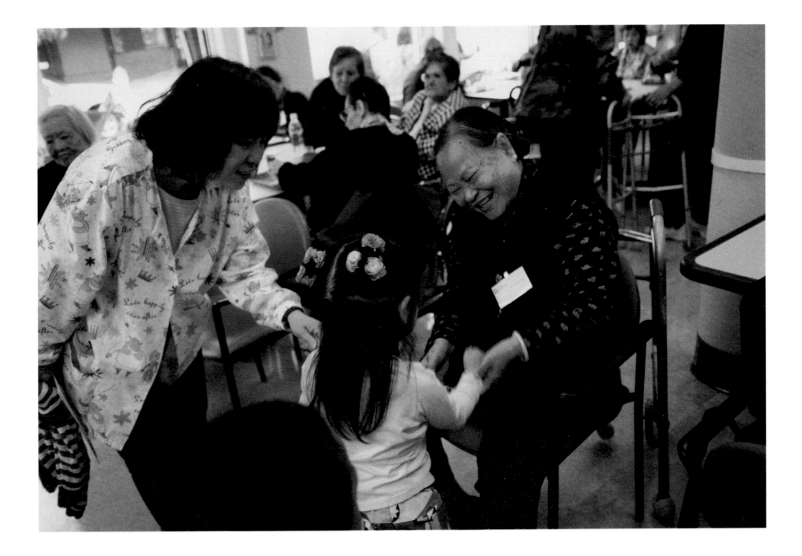

An estimated 12 million AIDS orphans are now struggling to survive in Africa, and Sister Magdaline Thiga, on the right, is one of the nurses helping them do that. As director of the Christian Women Works of Charity orphanage in Rongai, Kenya, she feeds, cares for, and educates abandoned children. With the help of female assistants, who know area residents, she also goes into the slum she serves to do AIDS testing.

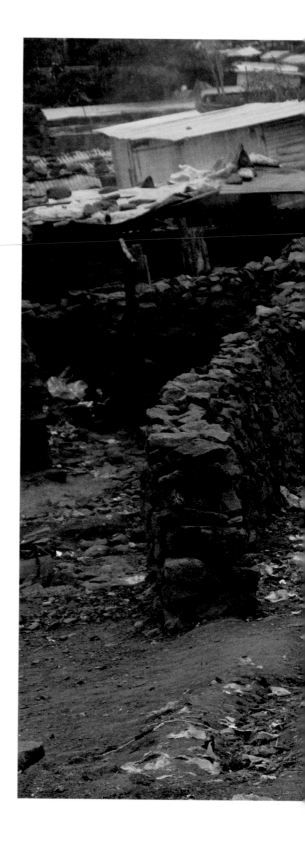

practitioner. Not long ago, she was appointed nursing and patient care supervisor at a large medical center in Minnesota. "I was surprised to discover how much I love doing this," said Toure-Keita. "Our patient and nursing populations are changing. We have many nurses from different countries and cultures working here now, but not many in administrative positions. I know I have a lot to offer, because I understand what it is like to be an immigrant," she said. Now the mother of four, she has just begun to pursue her master's degree in health care administration.

Nurses bring more than just their knowledge and expertise to these new fields. They also bring the practical problem-solving skills that nursing has long used to improvise creative solutions with limited resources, as well as the ability to organize and get things done. Many nurses are driven by the same sense of service and caring for humanity that attracted them to the profession in the first place. Some even bring the unique sense of humor that helps many nurses deal with the distress and suffering they often witness in their work.

Hob Osterlund is a pain and palliative care clinical nurse specialist in Hawaii. "My mother was a nurse, and I come from generations of missionaries and educators, so service has always been part of my genetics and culture," she said. Osterlund also has an infectious sense of humor. "I've always loved to joke. I've always had an eye and an ear out for the absurdities in life. The capacity for laughter is the capacity for intimacy. Especially in a hospital, laughter gives hope. It says things are okay, you're okay."

To give patients something to laugh about even in the darkest times, Osterlund created the Chuckle Channel, which provides comedy programming in hospitals. "A lot of patients wake up in the middle of the

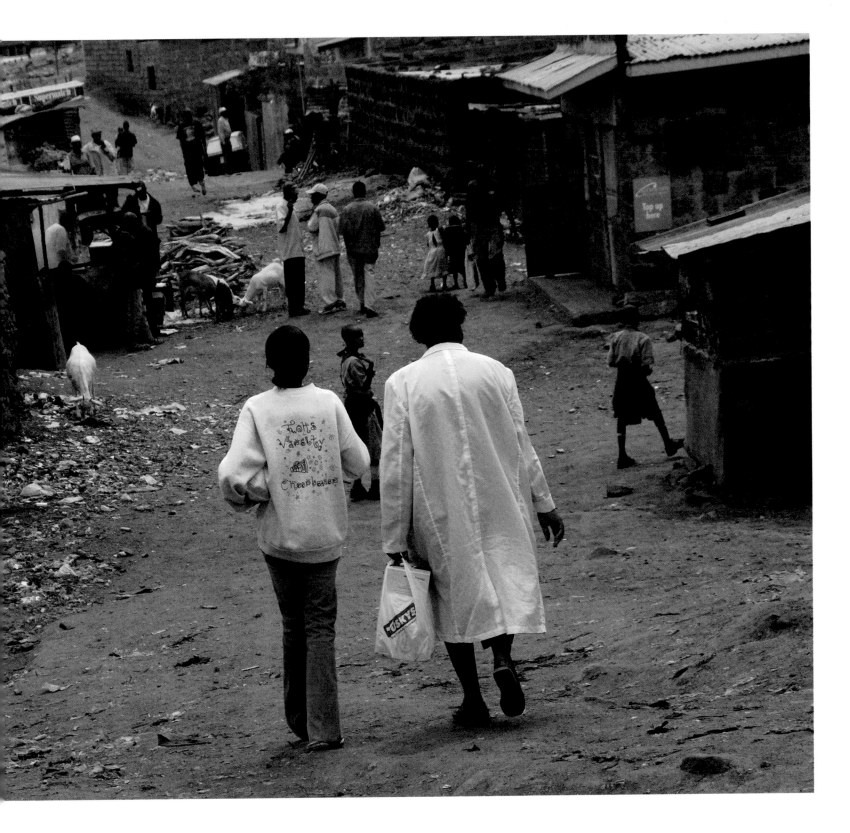

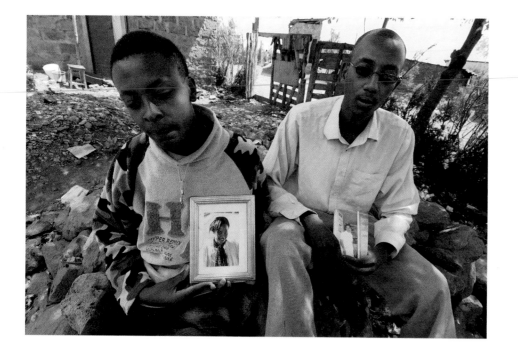

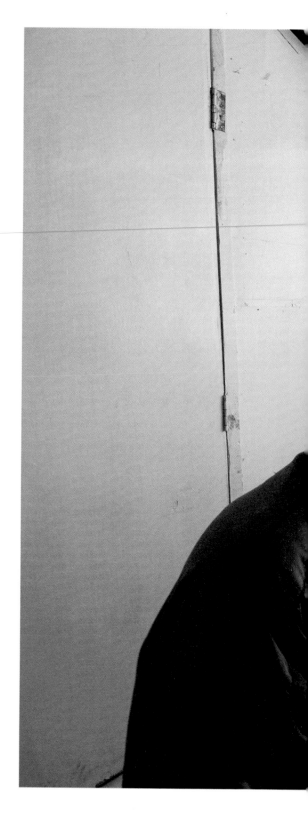

In her private clinic, Sister Magdaline offers nursing care to patients who can afford to pay (right). That gives her the economic freedom she needs to nurture AIDS orphans, like the two brothers above. The boys are luckier than most: Their mother—the nurse in the pictures they're holding—planned carefully for their future. She bought this small plot of land so that, after her death, her sons could rent out space to tenants for simple shelters and thus generate an income to live on. Nurses in unsafe working conditions are often at great risk of contracting AIDS and other diseases.

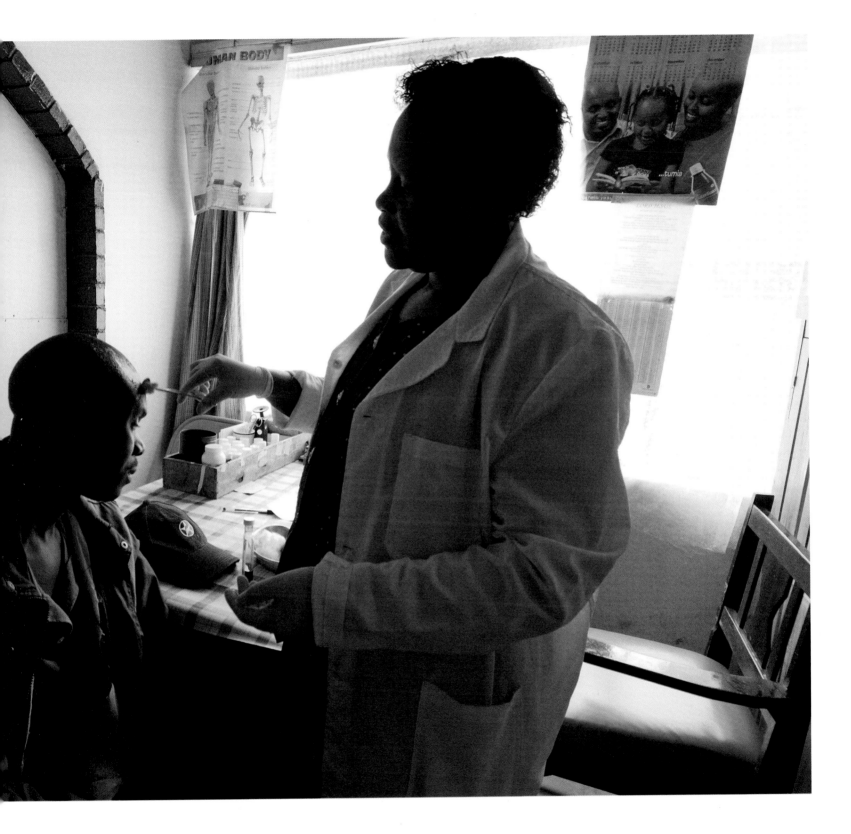

Concentrating on the job at hand, Kelly Moynes, a nursing student at Emory University, shaves one of the residents at a home run by the Missionaries of the Poor in Kingston, Jamaica. Each year, health professionals volunteer at the home for two weeks; many come away feeling that the experience has altered their lives forever.

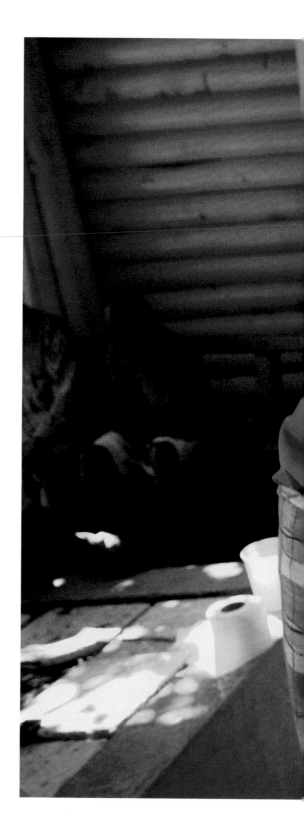

night, agitated or afraid. I wanted to give them something more than infomercials and bad news programs." She recently took on another role, too, that of nurse researcher, organizing a randomized study that will evaluate the effect of comedy on patients undergoing chemotherapy. She didn't stop there. Laughter, she decided, is something even nurses could use more of. And so Ivy Push, RN, was born. Osterlund's comic persona, Ivy has starred in two independent films and performed at countless medical conferences. "Us nurses are always in the middle," Ivy Push says in one skit, sitting in a utility closet at the hospital, the only place where she can find a little peace and quiet. "It's like holding two bare electric wires. One says, 'Do everything for everybody.' The other says, 'Cut costs every chance you can.' Hey, I'm getting shocked—and it's not therapy."

It's no surprise that nurses around the world, recognizing themselves in Ivy Push, RN, laugh out loud to hear her describe the joys and frustrations of nursing. Hob Osterlund, RN, who still practices as a nurse at the Queen's Medical Center in Honolulu, Hawaii, knows whereof she speaks.

RESEARCHERS, ADMINISTRATORS, ENTREPRENEURS, INVENTORS, COMEDIANS, public health experts, CEOs, policy makers, forensic investigators, —today's nurses are carrying the essential values of nursing into an ever widening field of professions. Their growing presence in so many areas offers new hope that we will find solutions to some of the most pressing problems facing us, from failing health care systems to the appalling inequities in access to basic care around the world. The new creative spirit in nursing has also inspired a new generation of young people to enter the profession.

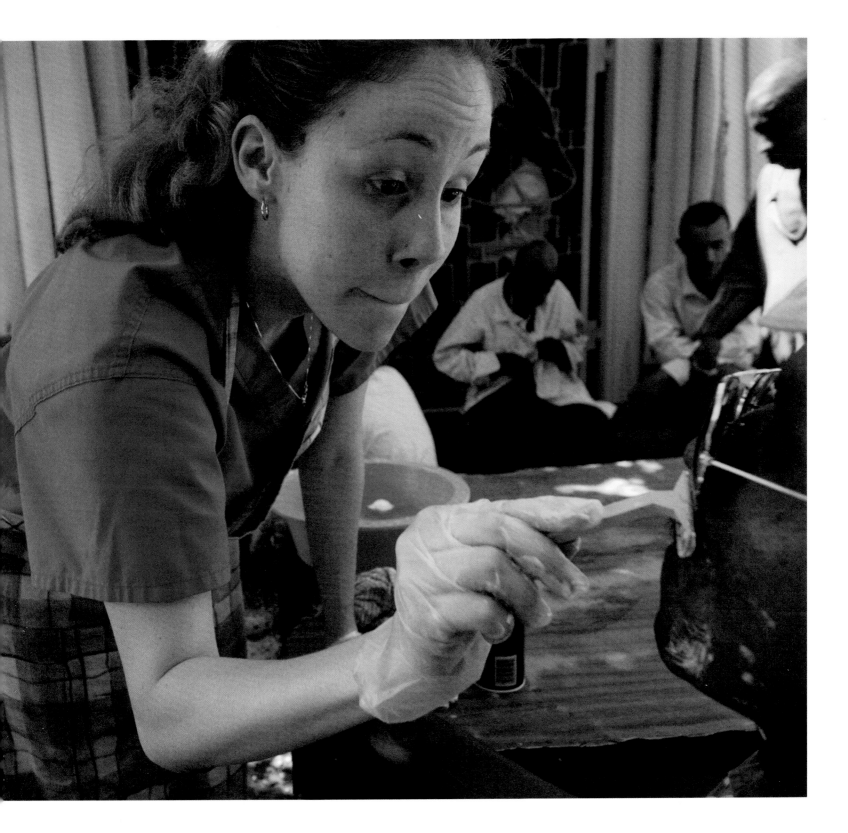

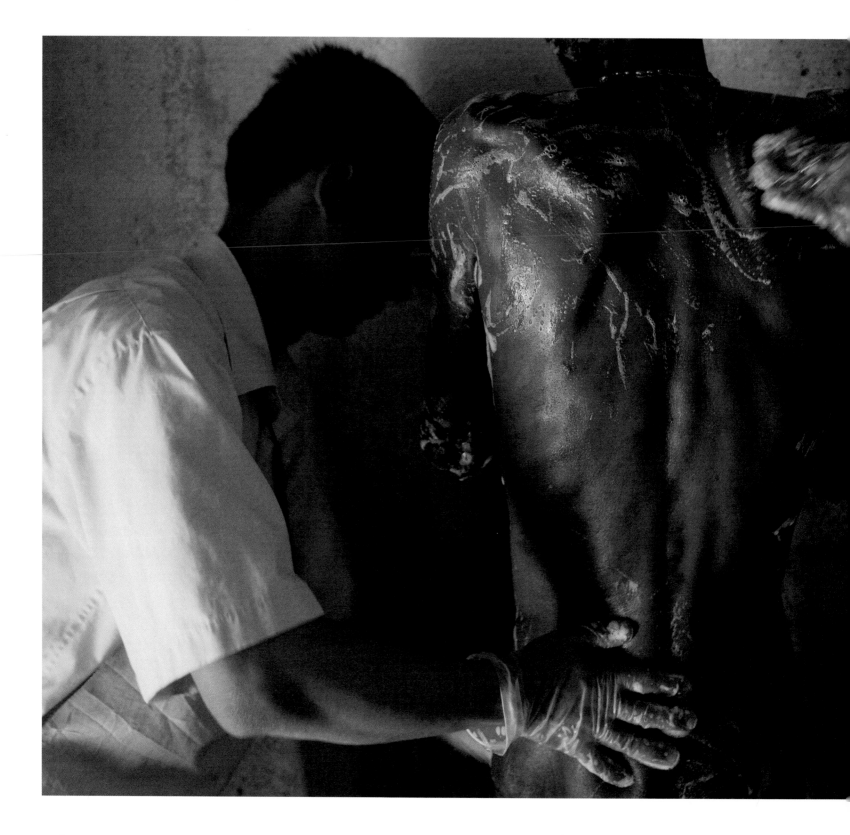

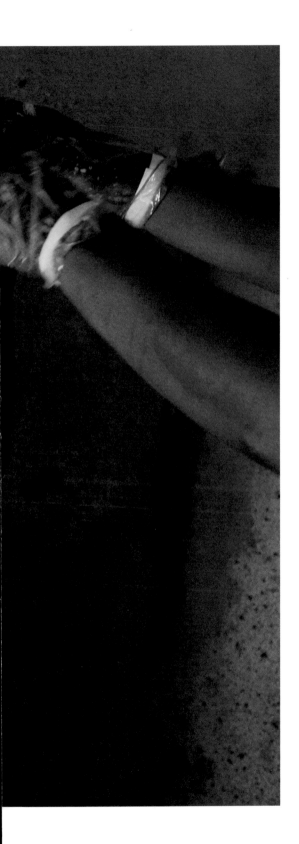

Brothers at Kingston's Missionaries of the Poor bathe a man with AIDS too weak to care for himself. Founded in Jamaica in 1981 as a new Catholic religious order, the Missionaries, some of whom are trained nurses, now maintain homes that serve people in need worldwide.

"I grew up thinking I'd be a pediatrician," said Anjli Aurora, whose family came to the U.S. from India. "But something about the medical profession wasn't in sync with who I was. I signed up for a class in women's health, taught by an incredible nurse midwife, and that was it. I'd found what I wanted to do." Now Aurora is a nursing and midwifery student at Nell Hodgson Woodruff School of Nursing at Emory University.

As a first-year nursing student, Aurora accompanied a group of other students to Kingston, Jamaica, to work with the Missionaries of the Poor, an international monastic order of brothers who care for the poor, destitute, homeless, and abandoned. In Jamaica, many of the 450 people they care for have HIV/AIDS. "All of them, no matter who they were, are treated with love and compassion. They are cared for by the brothers when no one else will touch them. Their lives are treated with dignity. I remember having the chance to go to a funeral of one of the residents who'd passed away. The brothers led a service in an almost empty church. They carried the coffin to the burial site. They dug the grave themselves. I'll never forget that. I don't know where my life will take me as a nurse midwife and nurse practitioner. But wherever that may be, I only hope to touch people's lives the way the brothers do every day."

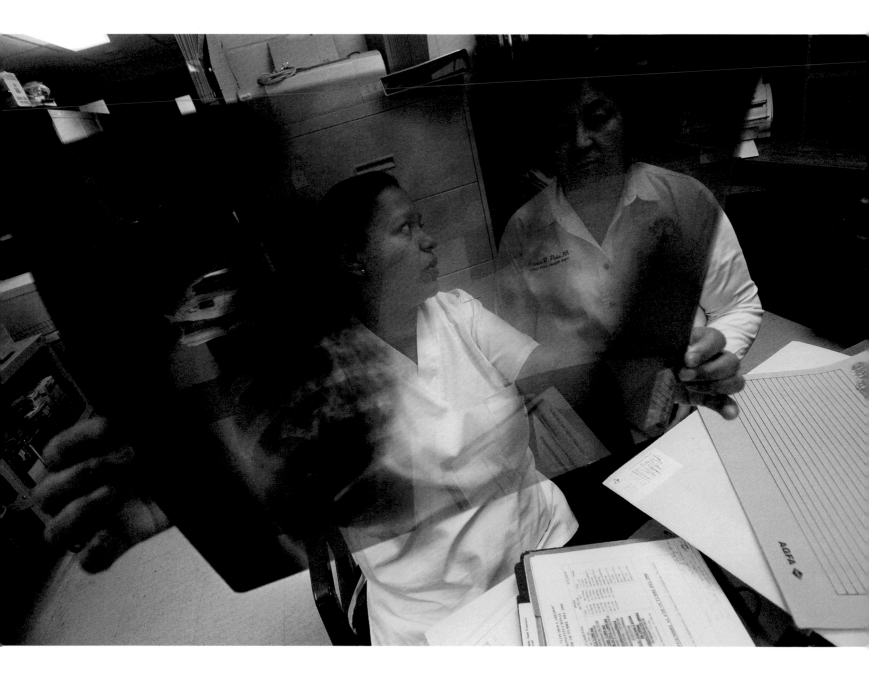

THREE   A CRUCIAL PARTNER

Popular images of nursing have long appealed to the heart—from wood engravings of Florence Nightingale holding her lamp as she makes her rounds to the World War II posters of a nurse with her hands outstretched, declaring, "Your Red Cross Needs You!"

Today, the image of nursing is much richer and more complex. Nurses are still motivated by the altruism of caring, of course. But they are also deeply engaged in the search for ways to improve the practice of nursing and to shape enlightened policies on behalf of the profession. Indeed, for almost a century and a half, nursing research has been building a solid base of scientific evidence that demonstrates the crucial importance of the profession and guides its practice.

Those efforts have done more than simply add to the body of medical science. They have helped extend the boundaries of health-related scientific enquiry into new areas. Guided by the profession's commitment to reach the most vulnerable and neglected and to offer comfort and compassion even when there may be no hope of a cure, nursing research has also helped preserve the human dimension in health studies in an era dominated by high-tech medicine. In doing so, it promises to change the face of health care.

Nursing transcends nationality: In Laredo, Texas, a Mexican and an American public health nurse involved in a cross-border health initiative confer over x-rays showing lungs infected with tuberculosis, a growing concern in this area.

Nursing research, like the modern profession of nursing itself, owes much to the lady with the lamp. When the 34-year-old Florence Nightingale, newly appointed superintendent of the Female Nursing Establishment of the English General Hospitals, arrived in Scutari, Turkey, during the Crimean War, she and her team of 38 nurses discovered a nightmarish scene: overcrowded barracks infested with rats and reeking of raw sewage and rotting food, clean water and even the most basic medical supplies in short supply. "There were no vessels for water or utensils of any kind," one of the nurses wrote. "No soap, towels, or clothes; no hospital clothes; the men lying in their uniforms, stiff with gore and covered with filth . . . ."

As the *Atlantic Monthly* reported in 1862, "Miss Nightingale and a large corps of assistants, attendants, and nurses, women of station and culture and women of hire, went to that terrible scene of misery and death, to aid in any measures that might be devised to alleviate the condition of the men. Great abuses and negligence were found; and the causes of disease were manifest, manifold, and needless. But a reform was at once instituted; great changes were made in the general management of the camp and hospitals and in the condition of soldiers."

Nightingale went further. In 1858, she published an 800-page report on her experiences, using statistics to argue her case for improving sanitation and medical care in military and civilian hospitals. The death rate when she arrived at Scutari was almost 43 percent. Six months later the rate had fallen to just 2.2 percent—providing convincing evidence that her methods worked.

Day of the Dead brings nurses working in Laredo across the Mexican border to Nuevo Laredo. They've come out of respect and support for a nursing colleague, who is placing the traditional flowers on the grave of a loved one.

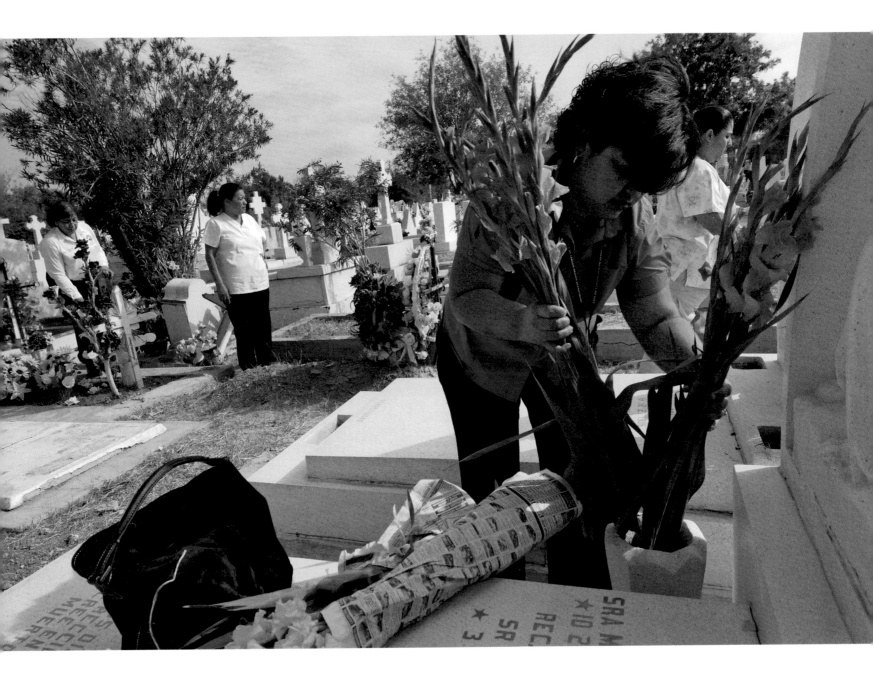

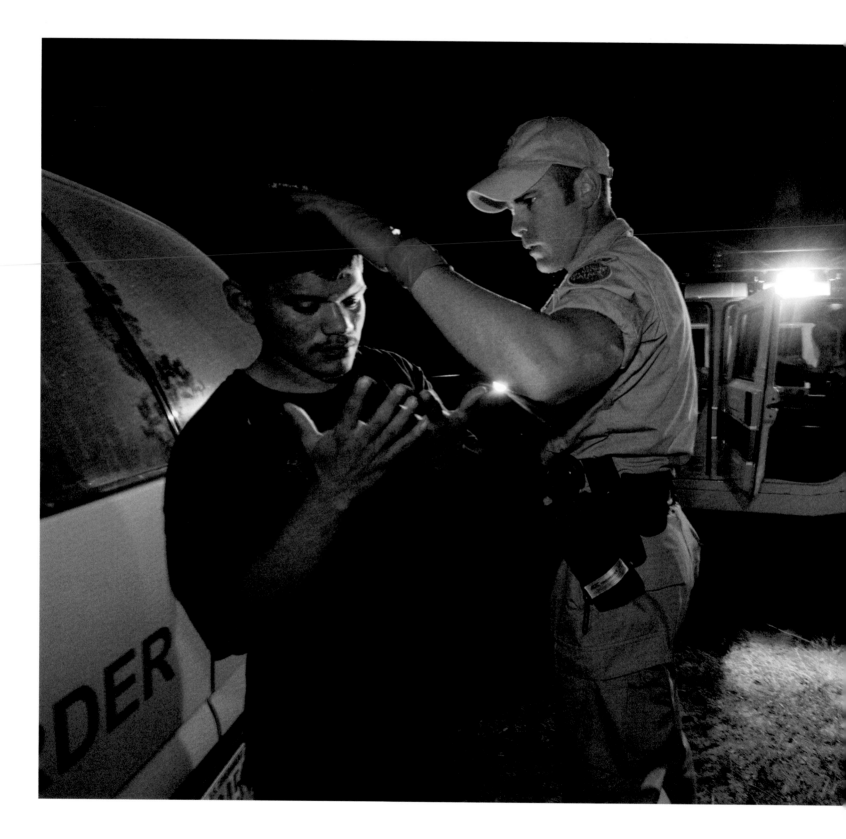

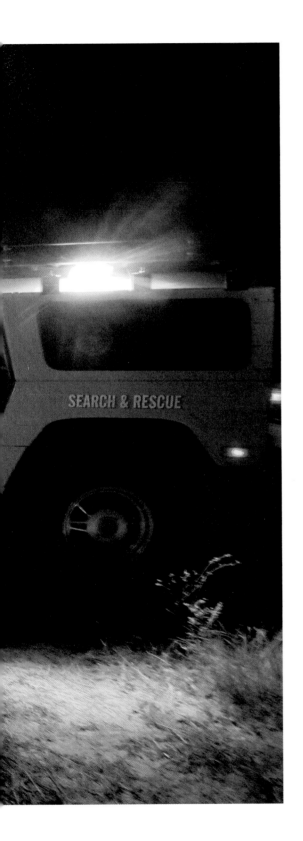

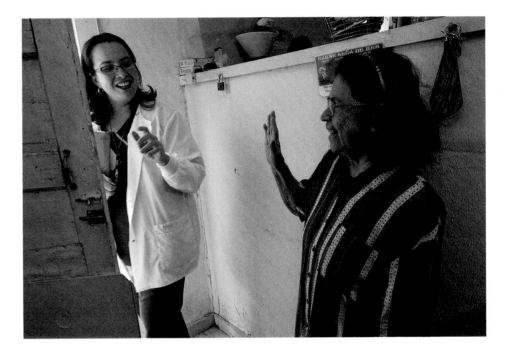

Border patrol agent and first responder Jason Wood has to have a medic's skills to do his job. Besides removing cactus spines (left), he treats more serious injuries and ailments in the travelers he apprehends attempting to cross into the U.S. illegally. Public health nurses in the border area are often faced with chronic health problems. The nurse above has just administered TB drugs to a patient in Laredo. Using DOT—"directly observed therapy"—the nurse visits the home and watches as the patient takes all medications, a critical component in combating tuberculosis.

Nightingale's detailed analysis gave birth to the field of nursing research, which gradually came into its own as an independent field of investigation. In 1899, the International Council of Nurses was founded by a small group of nurses from Britain and the U.S., the first international association of health professionals in the world. Now based in Geneva, Switzerland, the ICN membership roster includes nursing associations from 132 countries. One of its key missions is still the advancement of research in nursing practice. In 1900, the first issue of the *American Journal of Nursing* was published. Two World Wars would prove an important testing ground, a time when nurses took on new responsibilities, gained greater respect, and extended their expertise. In 1922, Sigma Theta Tau, the honor society of nursing, was founded to promote nursing leadership and research. In 1952, the journal *Nursing Research* began publication, introducing a new forum for the exchange and evaluation of ideas. Three years later, the U.S. federal government created a national Division of Nursing at the Health Resources and Services Administration. One of its signal contributions was the creation of a doctorate degree in nursing, which greatly expanded the opportunities for nurses in both academics and research. The National Center for Nursing Research at the National Institutes of Health came into being in 1985. Eight years later it was elevated to the status of an institute, in recognition of the central role of nursing research in medicine.

Meanwhile, around the world institutions dedicated to nursing research were taking root. Britain's Royal College of Nursing commenced in 1975, the Japanese Academy of Nursing Science in 1981. In 1992, the World

Clearly, the involvement of nurses and midwives in pregnancies and births dramatically improves both the mother's and child's chances of survival and health.

Health Organization created the Global Advisory Group on Nursing and Midwifery. For the first time, the impact of nursing and midwifery would be acknowledged by health professionals as a key factor in international health goals and policies.

LIKE THE PROFESSION IT REPRESENTS, NURSING RESEARCH HAS OFTEN focused on ways to expand access to health care and improve the quality of care, especially for people who have been neglected. It's no coincidence that when the National Center for Nursing Research became an institute, one of its first major studies looked at preventing high blood pressure in young African American men, a population at very high risk of this serious condition and one that had been largely neglected by earlier research. As former U.S. Surgeon General Richard H. Carmona, himself both a registered nurse and a physician, pointed out in 2003: "This was the first time that many of the young men had ever been contacted by any health care organization or offered any preventive health care."

In another reflection of the enduring values of the profession, nurse researchers have taken special interest in care at both the beginning and the end of life, when people are at their most vulnerable. After crusading to improve care for pregnant women and families in New York City and Washington, D.C., for instance, nursing leader Ruth Lubic went on to conduct groundbreaking research on the benefits of birthing centers staffed by nurses and midwives. The landmark 1989 National Birth Center Study, which looked at 11,814 women cared for at 84 freestanding birthing centers, found that these women and their infants suffered

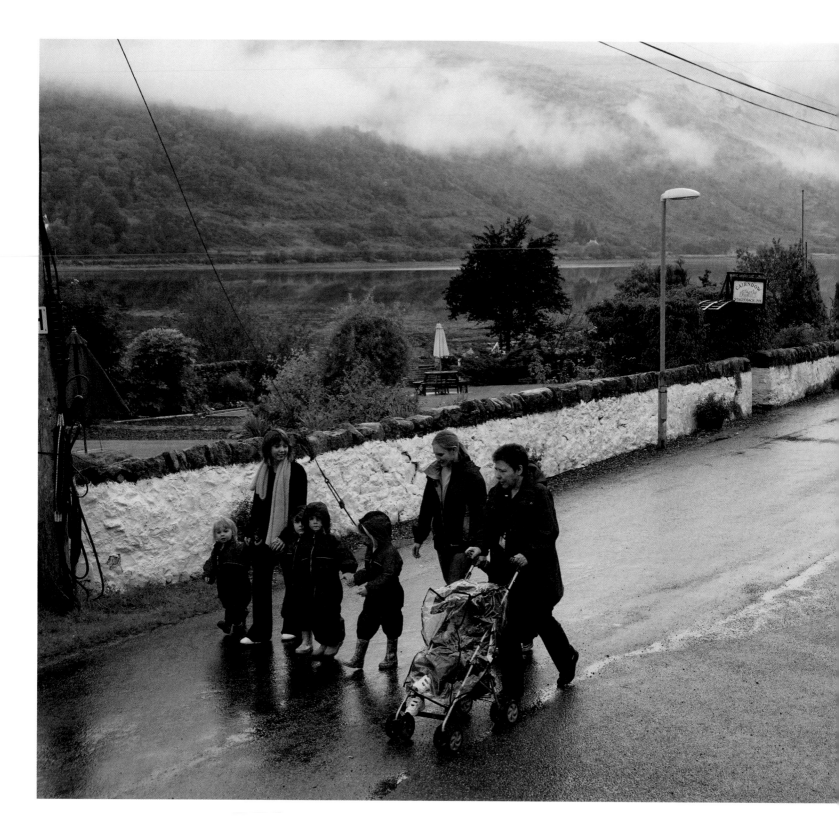

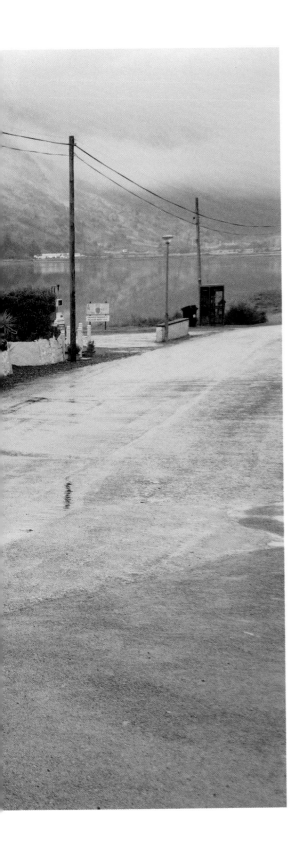

In the scattered towns of the Scottish Highlands, community health nurses serve as primary care providers for the entire family, thanks to a pilot program begun by the National Health Service. Living in the community, getting to know its rhythms and the individual concerns of its citizens enable these providers to offer an engaged, personal level of care.

no maternal deaths and a rate of neonatal deaths comparable to the lowest rates found in hospital obstetrics units. Significantly, women cared for at birthing centers were half as likely as hospitalized women to have cesarean sections—powerful evidence that the centers kept mothers and babies healthy while also saving on health care costs. Following in Lubic's footsteps, researchers at Florida International University's School of Nursing showed in 1991 that women with high-risk pregnancies who received home visits from advanced-practice nurses suffered fewer miscarriages, were less likely to be hospitalized, and gave birth to babies who were less likely to have to spend time in the hospital. Although the home-visit program included only 85 women, it eliminated the need for more than 750 days in the hospital and saved $2.5 million.

In parts of the world with only the most basic health care, maternal health programs like these also save lives. A 2005 study by researchers at the Society for Education, Action and Research in Community Health in Gadchiroli, India, demonstrated that a program in which village health workers made prenatal, home-birthing, and neonatal visits to rural women reduced the risk of infant and maternal deaths by almost 50 percent. In Gambia, a collaboration between nurse midwives and traditional birth attendants helped reduce maternal mortality rates from 700 to only 130 deaths for every 100,000 live births. A comprehensive family health program in Sri Lanka that included community midwives and skilled birth attendants helped slash maternal mortality deaths from 520 to only 66 per 100,000 live births. Clearly, the involvement of nurses and midwives in pregnancies and births dramatically improves both the mother's and child's chances of survival and health.

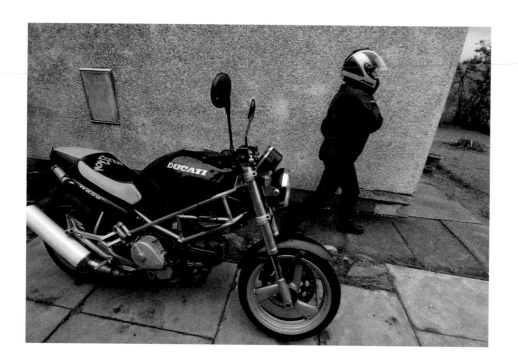

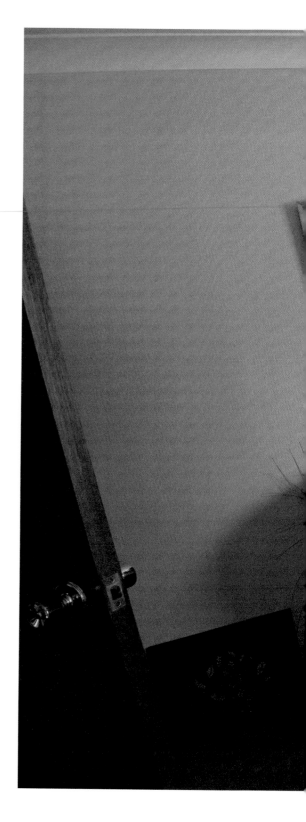

No longer able to leave his home in Inveraray, Scotland, an elderly man still receives the medical attention he needs, thanks to Ann Templeton, the family nurse for the community. Like the long-gone—and much missed—country doctor, Ann knows her patients and their home situations well and is always there for them. When she has a bit of time to herself, she and her husband like to bike (above) through the Scottish Highlands.

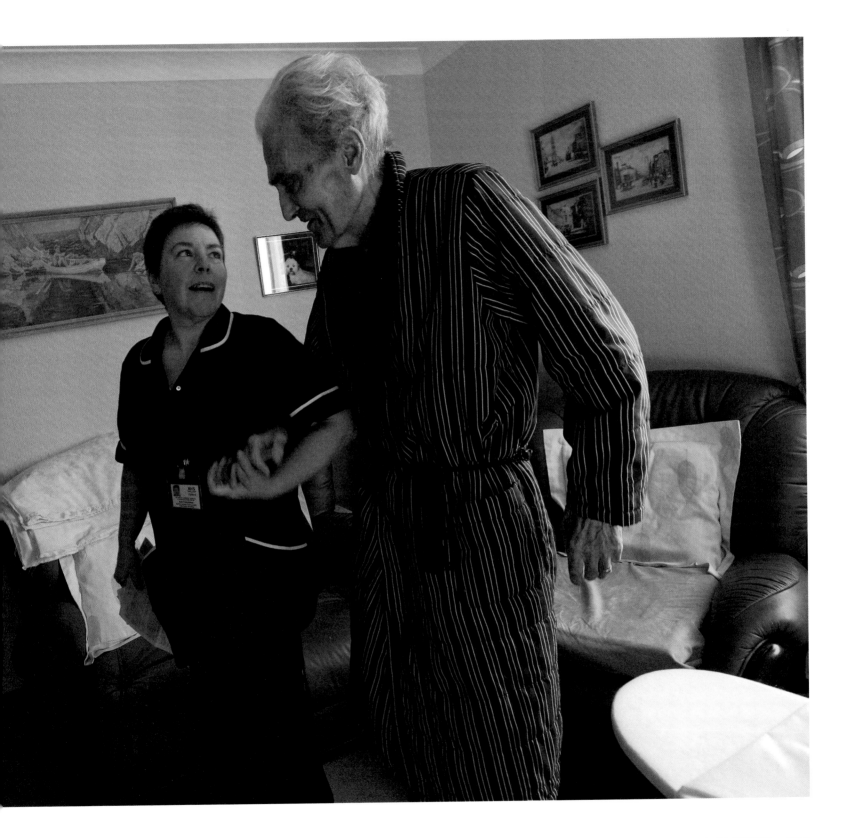

GIVING MEANING TO HUMAN LIFE, ESPECIALLY IN THE FACE OF ILLNESS AND death, is equally a part of the mission of nursing—central to the profession's commitment to offering comfort and care for patients who can't be cured. Acknowledging that sacred role, the U.S. National Institute for Nursing Research was directed in 1997 to lead collaborative research nationwide in the field of pain and palliative medicine. Nursing researchers immediately launched a wide range of studies to explore the current state of end-of-life care and to chart ways to improve it. Instead of hard numbers, many of these investigations used information gleaned from listening to patients and their families describe their experiences, another reflection of the spirit of nursing. The findings have inspired new approaches to hospice care that are designed to allow dying patients, their loved ones, and their caregivers to find not only comfort but also dignity and meaning in death. The campaign to improve end-of-life care is spreading around the world. In Uganda, for instance, palliative care training is now part of the curriculum at both medical and nursing schools. The country recently amended its laws so that nurses who complete special training in palliative medicine can prescribe narcotic pain medications.

The values of nursing inform research in other ways, too. Nurses have always been committed to treating people as whole human beings, not just bodies. So it's only natural that nursing researchers should take the lead in the field of holistic medicine, which explores the way mind, body, and spirit influence health and well-being. Nursing is also at the forefront of investigating ways to improve preventive health measures in communities. To that end, nurses themselves have served as the study

Nurses have always been committed to treating people as whole human beings, not just bodies.

group in the long-running epidemiologic investigation called the Nurses Health Study. For more than three decades, some 122,000 U.S. nurses have participated in the study, designed first to look at the consequences of oral contraceptive use and later expanded to include the impact of diet and lifestyle on health. The study has generated hundreds of research papers, on everything from the cardiovascular benefits of whole grains to the impact of walking and other forms of exercise on health and longevity. In a landmark 2000 study based on data from the Nurses Health Study, researchers at Boston's Brigham and Women's Hospital and Harvard Medical School demonstrated that more than 80 percent of cases of cardiovascular disease can be avoided through healthier lifestyle choices.

NURSING PRACTICE ITSELF HAS COME UNDER THE RESEARCH MICROSCOPE, as the profession puts its methods to the test in an effort to improve care. Those efforts took on new urgency in 2000, when the Institute of Medicine, part of the National Academy of Sciences, published a groundbreaking report called *To Err Is Human: Building a Safer Health System*. The report presented shocking evidence that as many as 98,000 hospitalized Americans die every year not through illness or disease but as a result of medical errors—more deaths than result from motor vehicle accidents, breast cancer, or AIDS. In a follow-up report published in 2004, the Institute of Medicine singled out nursing care as the crucial agent for change.

With good reason. The follow-up report, titled *Keeping Patients Safe: Transforming the Work Environment of Nurses,* noted that, "When people

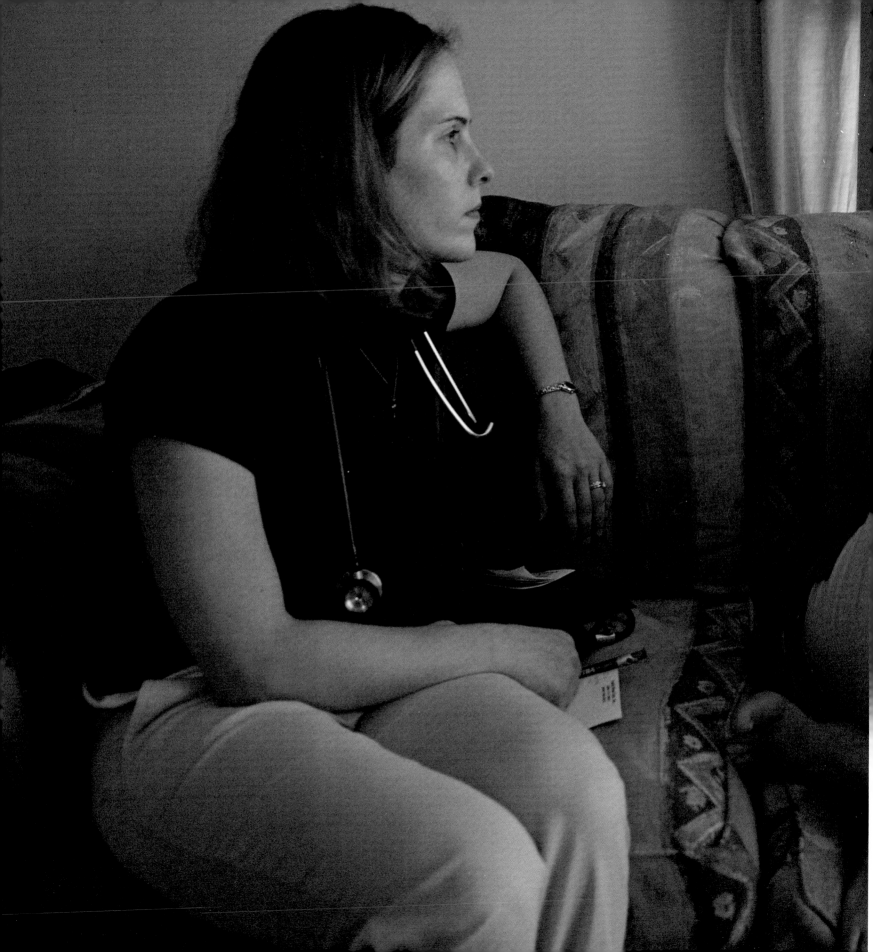

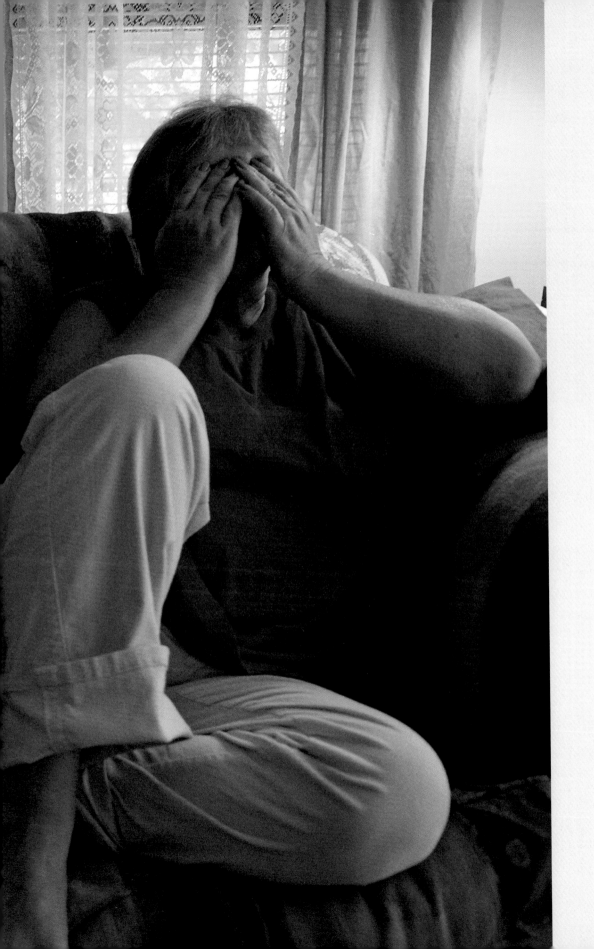

FRONTIER NURSING

Life has always been a challenge in southeastern Kentucky, where few jobs and little money can make it hard even to afford indoor plumbing or gas for your car. Sarah Noggle knows this area and these people firsthand. As a family nurse practitioner, she visits them in their homes if they can't get to the clinic she helps run in Asher. Poor diet and lack of both exercise and funds for medicine or doctor visits

Nurse practitioner Sarah Noggle trains a kind but professional eye on a patient who struggles with psychiatric problems. Many of her patients are isolated in their rural homes, so Sarah makes regular house calls.

all contribute to physical and emotional problems in these hardscrabble Appalachian hills.

"A vast majority of the patients we see have diabetes, a complex disease. And they have high blood pressure, high cholesterol, elevated risk of heart disease, and other complications. They need a lot of care," says Sarah, who is with Frontier Nursing Service, the organization founded in the 1920s by Mary Breckenridge. Much expanded, FNS now provides affordable, comprehensive family care at clinics and in homes in this part of Kentucky. "In a community like this, the most effective thing we can do is help empower people to do for themselves," Sarah says, "to encourage them to take their health seriously and give them some simple advice on what to do."

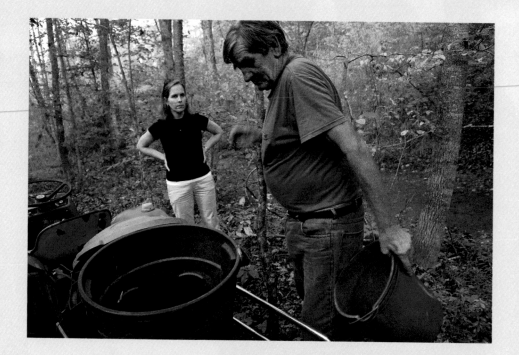

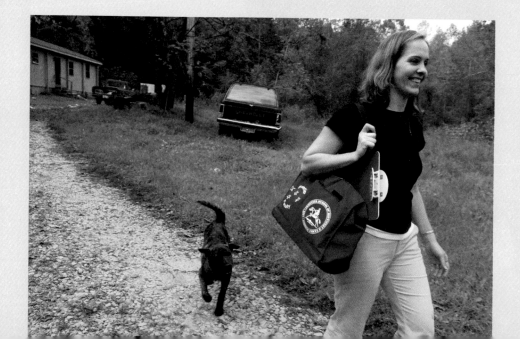

Staving off disaster, Sarah and a colleague (below) realize that a man who has come to their clinic with chest pains is having a heart attack. Living conditions here in southeastern Kentucky hardly contribute to health: Most of the homes Sarah visits are simple and remote (bottom); some lack indoor plumbing, so owners have to cart water from nearby creeks (left).

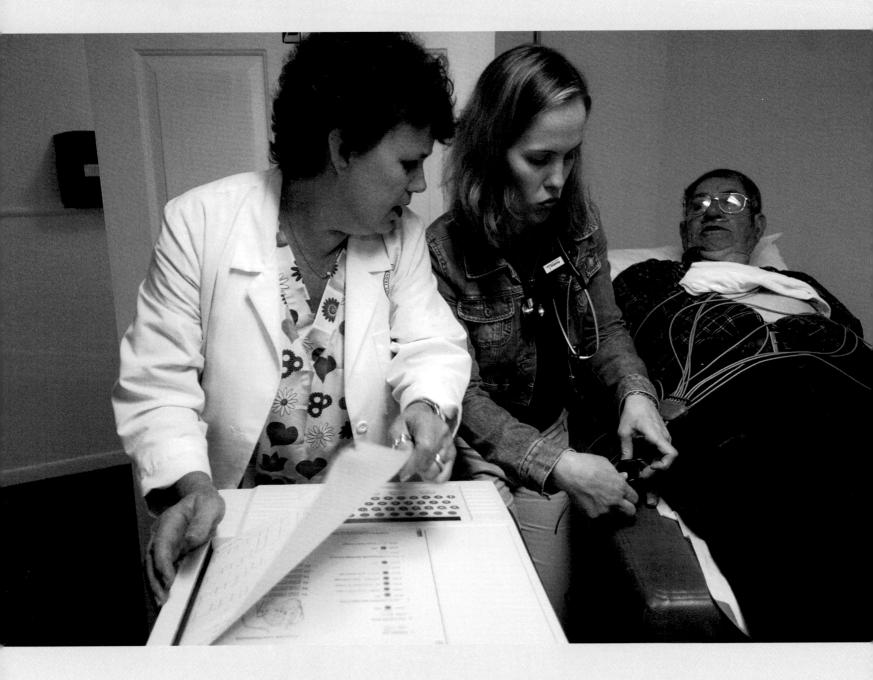

In Ethiopia's capital of Addis Ababa, many houses are no more than walls constructed of cardboard and scrap materials—rough places to be dying of AIDS. Sister Yewaganesh, a nurse with the Hiwot HIV/AIDS Prevention, Care, and Support Organization, ministers to these patients in their homes. The organization, founded by another nurse, is community based and funded by local donations.

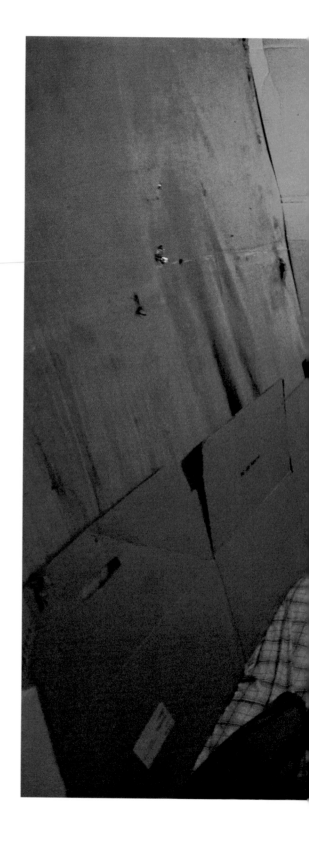

are hospitalized, in a nursing home, having a baby, or learning to manage a chronic condition in their own home—at some of their most vulnerable moments—nurses are the health care providers they are most likely to encounter; spend the greatest amount of time with; and, along with other health care providers, depend on for their recovery."

And often for their safety. Errors in prescribing or filling medications are a leading cause of harm to hospitalized patients. An influential 1995 investigation found that nurses were responsible for catching almost nine out of ten medication errors made by physicians, pharmacies, and others. Their vigilance saves untold numbers of lives.

Yet even as the first Institute of Medicine report was published, nursing care was under threat as hospitals and other health care facilities sought to balance budgets by cutting staffs. With administrators wielding the knife, researchers debated the most cost-effective ratios of nurses to patients. That debate proved to be more than an academic exercise. Analyzing data from 168 hospitals and more than 232,000 hospitalized patients, a research team from the Center for Health Outcomes and Policy Research at the University of Pennsylvania found that for each additional patient a nurse has to care for—and thus the less time they can spend with each patient—mortality rates climb 7 percent. When the ratio increases from one nurse per four patients to one per eight, overall mortality soars 31 percent.

The same pattern shows up in hospitals around the world. In 2007, researchers at the Florence Nightingale School of Nursing and Midwifery at King's College London reported that overall mortality rates were 26 percent higher in hospitals where nurses had to care for the

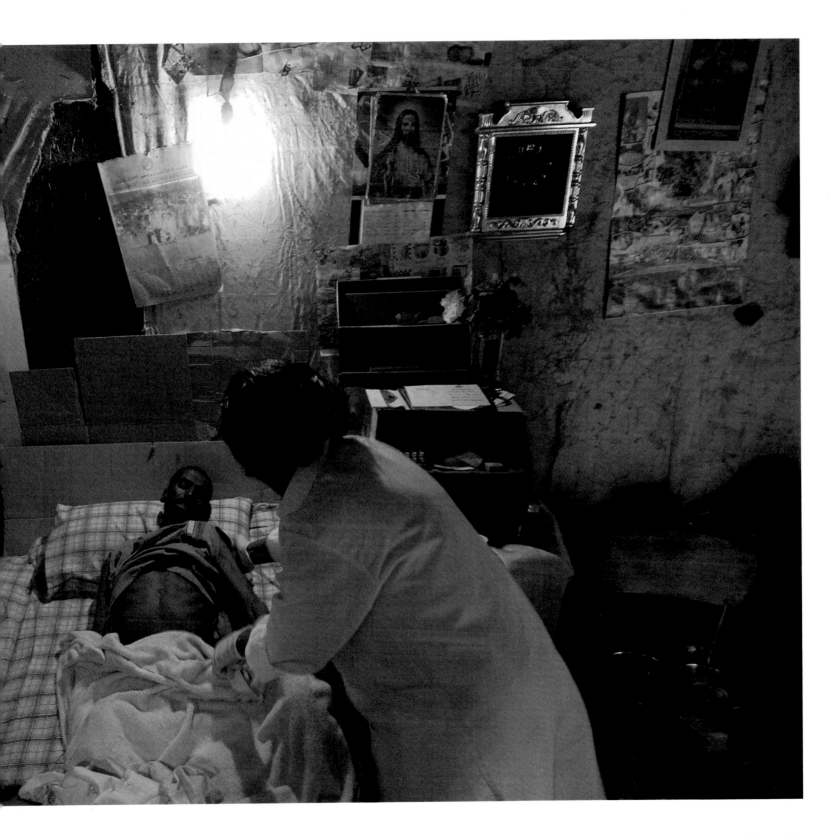

Coffee ceremonies—cherished Ethiopian traditions that involve roasting, grinding, and brewing—have been put to good use by AIDS outreach educators. They use the ceremonies as a way to gather neighbors at a local home and explain to them how to prevent and treat the disease.

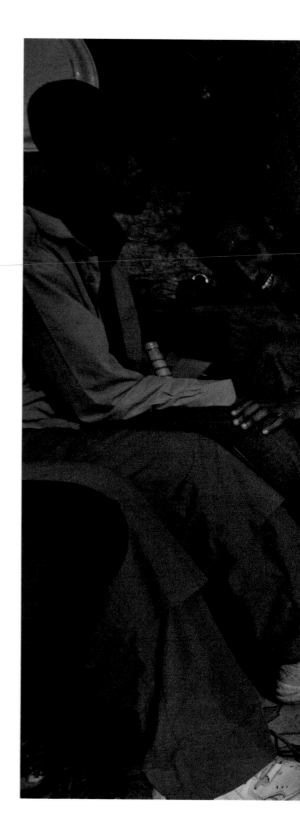

largest number of patients. In an examination of 75 acute-care hospital units in Ontario, Canada, researchers found that a 10 percent increase in the number of registered nurses at a hospital resulted in six fewer deaths per thousand patients admitted. In these and many other studies, fewer nurses on staff have consistently been associated with higher rates of what researchers call "failure to rescue." When nursing staffs are overstretched, in other words, patients who suffer cardiac arrest or a precipitous drop in blood pressure are more likely to die. Hospitalized patients are also more likely to suffer complications. Using data from 799 hospitals and more than five million patients, researchers at the Harvard School of Public Health in Boston reported in 2002 that lower nursing staff levels were consistently associated with higher patient risk of developing pneumonia, upper gastro-intestinal bleeding, and urinary tract infections. In one analysis, having more registered nurses on hand was associated with as much as a 12 percent reduction in such complications. Other studies have linked inadequate nursing levels to other serious complications, including collapsed lungs, pressure ulcers, and falls.

Findings like these are important beyond simply proving the benefits of nursing care. They play a crucial role in informing the debate over ways to allocate scarce health care resources and to promote more enlightened health care policies. In both the developed and the developing world, these findings argue for programs that extend access to care by supporting the work of nurses and midwives. They make the case for reorganizing the workplace in hospitals, nursing homes, and other health care facilities to enhance nursing efficiency and improve patient

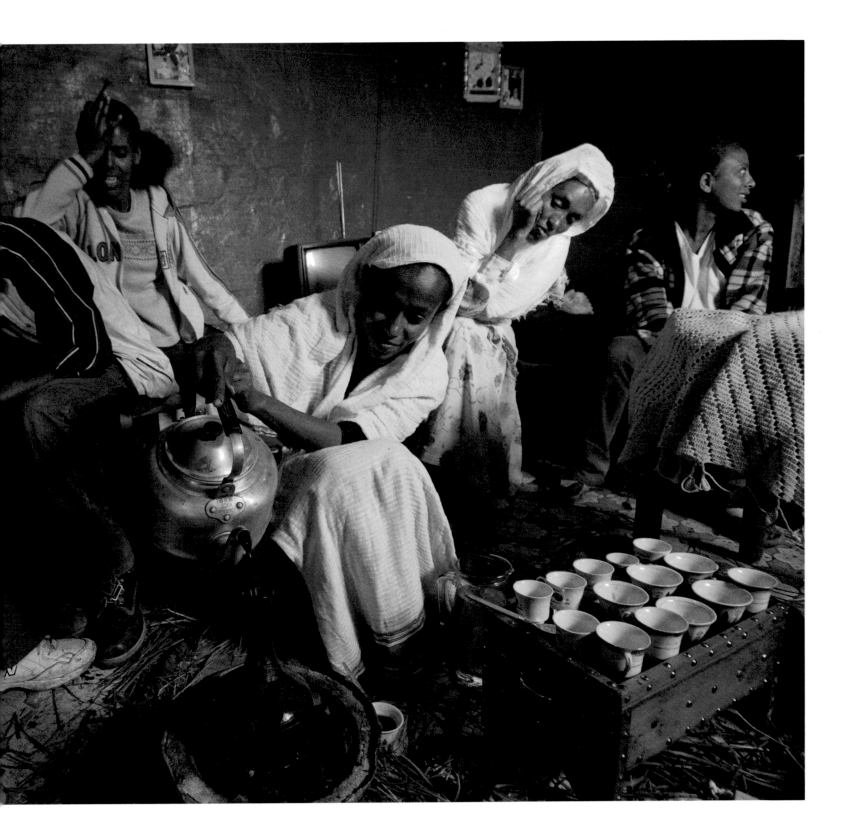

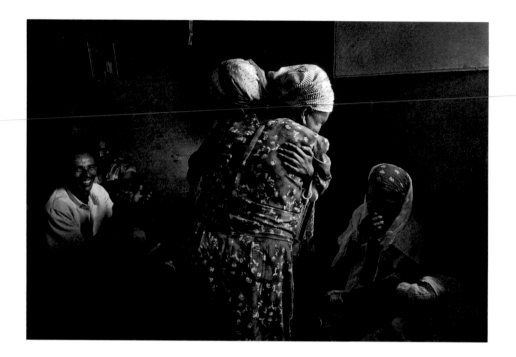

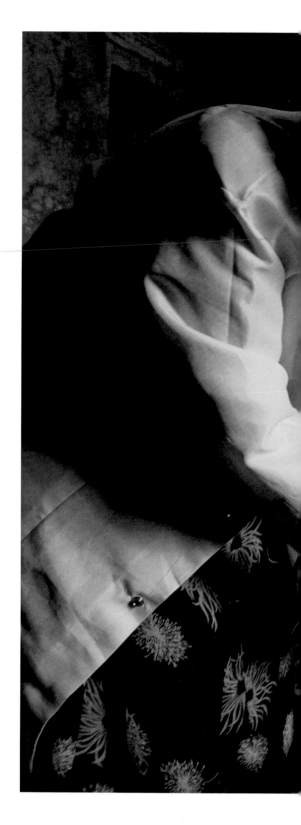

After attending a coffee ceremony at the home of an Addis Ababa neighbor, two women part friends (above). Before the ceremony began, they had reconciled their differences over an ongoing dispute. Such ceremonies are meant to release tensions and generate positive feelings. They create an open, accepting forum for AIDS educators to destigmatize the disease and encourage community support for those who have it. Right: Volunteers-in-training, like the young man holding medicine bottles, often accompany Sister Yewaganesh on her rounds. If they show potential, she recommends them for more formal training.

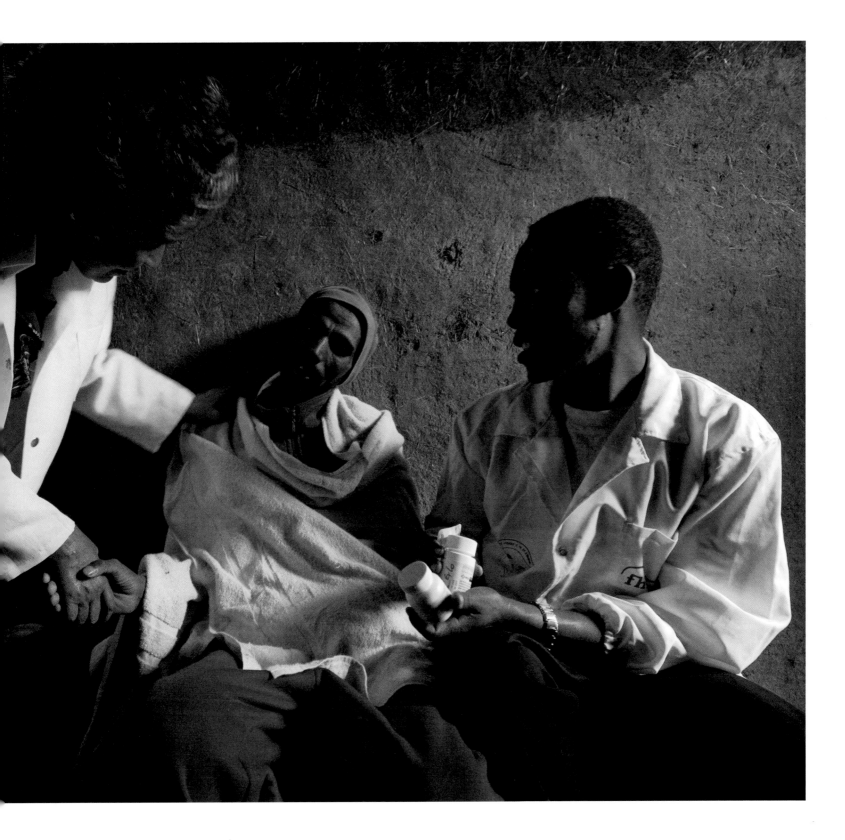

safety. They offer compelling evidence that when nurses are given more autonomy, patients are healthier and lives are saved. Most important of all, they prove that nurses, far from being an expense that can be cut to balance the budget, are a crucial and cost-effective investment in the health of individuals, families, and communities.

AS IMPORTANT AS STATISTICS AND RESEARCH FINDINGS ARE, THEY TELL ONLY part of the story. Much of what nurses do—whether as village health workers in Kenya or midwives in Kentucky, geriatric registered nurses in an Australian long-term care facility in Sydney, or school nurses in an inner city school in the Bronx—can't be captured in charts and figures. The work of nurses is literally beyond measure. Nurses may begin by treating individuals, but they often end up caring for whole communities, offering not just a better chance for a healthier life but something just as precious: hope.

That's what Sarah Noggle loves best about her work. A family nurse practitioner in Asher, Kentucky, Sarah sees most patients at a small clinic in town, but she also makes frequent home visits to those who can't drive or can't afford the price of gas. "This is a very rural area, with remote towns that are just a handful of houses," she explained. "By going into people's homes, you can see firsthand how they live. You can look at what's in their medicine cabinet and in their pantry. By becoming part of the community, you know that skim milk costs an extra twenty cents at the IGA, which is a lot for some people. You know that many people can't read, so you take extra time to go over the directions for taking a medication. There's a lot of poverty here, so you always try to find the

Well-known and well liked, Sister Yewaganesh is greeted by two teenage girls who live in the community she serves. Once a government employee, she retired early so she could help with the AIDS epidemic ravaging Addis Ababa.

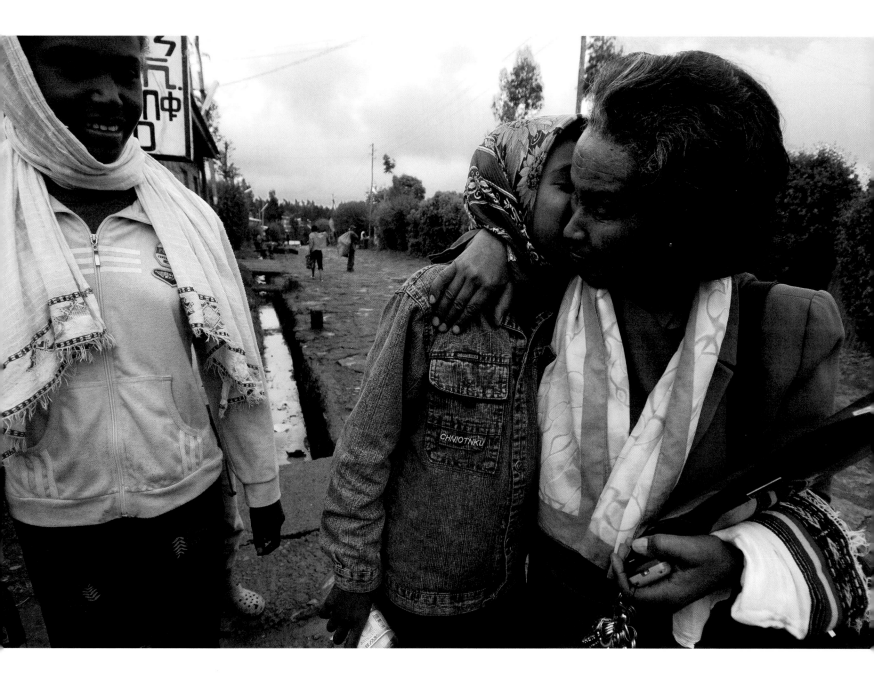

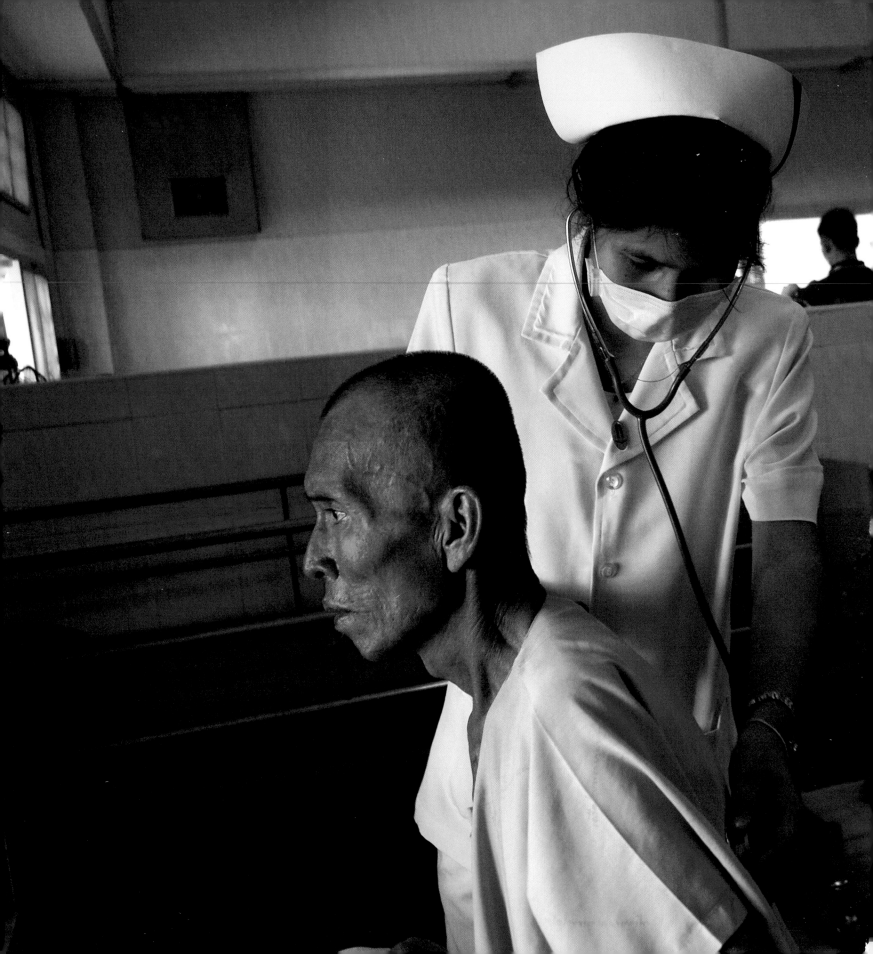

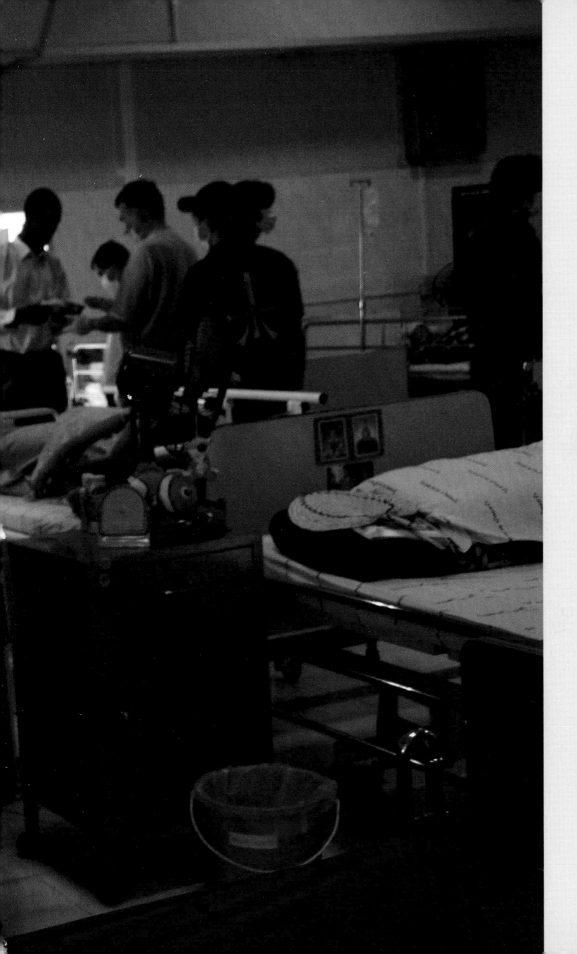

LOVING CARE

"Compassion and love are not mere luxuries," the Dalai Lama has said. "They are fundamental to the continued survival of our species."

Those basic Buddhist tenets are put into practice at the Wat Pra Bahpnampu Buddhist Monastery outside Lop Buri City, Thailand. A hospice adjacent to the temple is devoted to treating those who are dying of AIDS with compassion, love, and the spiritual and medical

Nurse Wiliawan Khantiwongse juggles many duties, from supervising the overworked staff of practical nurses on her ward to caring for patients.

attention they need to ease their pain.

Supported by donations, the Buddhist hospice faces challenges. Understaffed by about 50 percent of what is needed, it has to deal not only with the debilitating effects of AIDS but with the complications brought on by a weakened immune system—notably the specter of TB. Many patients here suffer from both.

Hospice nurses offer basic care, to keep patients as comfortable and pain-free as possible through medications, hygiene, and diet.

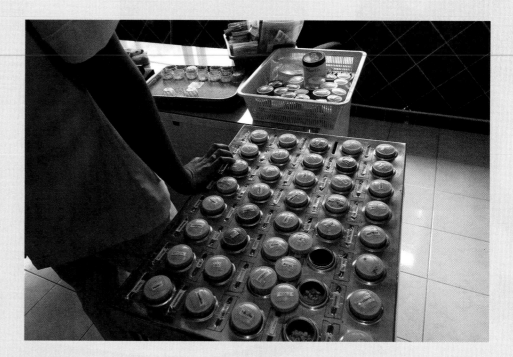

Spiritual ministrations are a critical part of care in the hospice, and the
Buddhist monk below visits fellow patients daily. Diagnosed with AIDS
himself, he came to the hospice for treatment and became a monk.
Patients also receive the antiretroviral cocktail of drugs and vitamins (left)
that help control their condition.

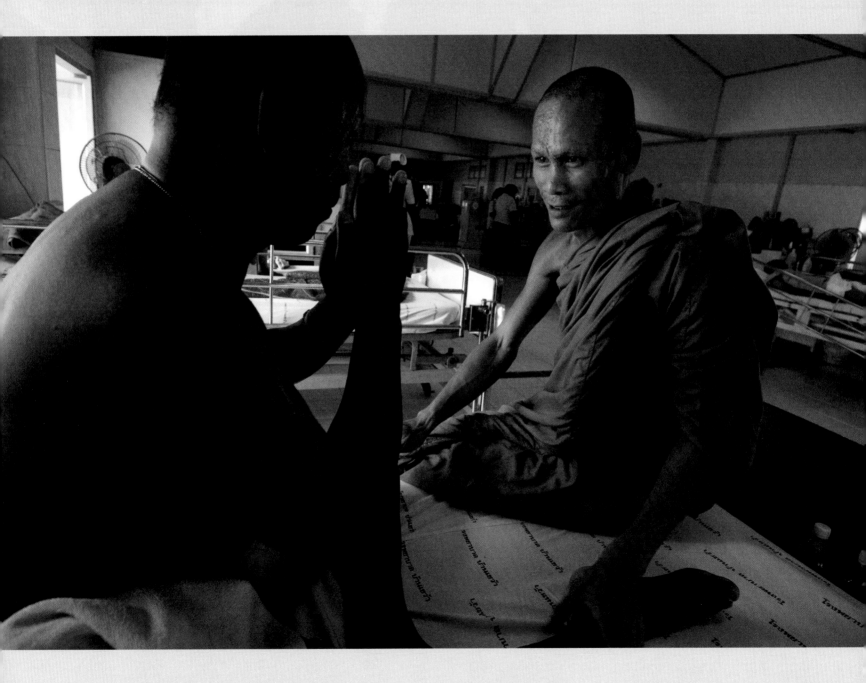

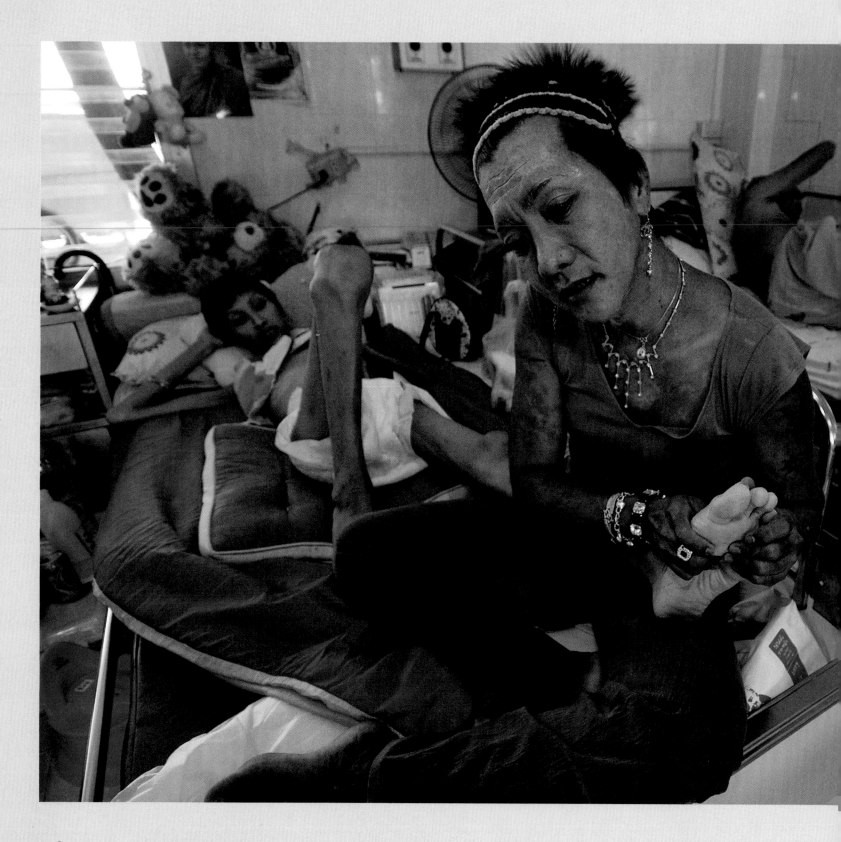

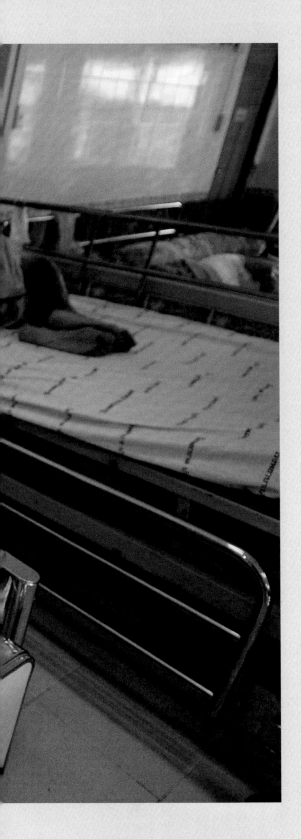

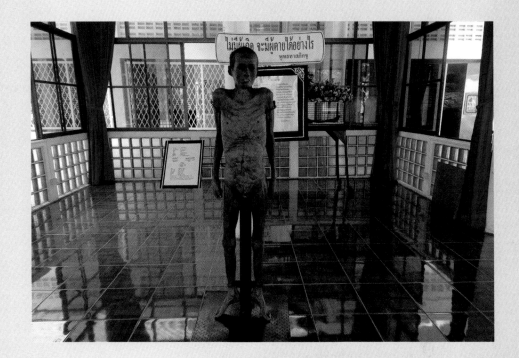

With a keen compassion for the pains of others, hospice patients offer simple kindnesses to one another (left). The man on the right, once a transvestite performer, gives another resident a foot massage. On public display, the cadaver (above) of a former AIDS patient draws several thousand visitors a week—their donations provide an important source of financial support to the hospice, and the display also serves as a warning about the ravages of AIDS.

most cost-effective treatment, because if something is too expensive, people won't use it."

Aware that many children were falling through the cracks, Sarah helped start a school-based clinic where she routinely diagnoses asthma, vision problems, and infections that might otherwise have gone unnoticed. One problem that's all too obvious, here and in many parts of the world, is obesity. "So we're looking at starting an aerobics class at the community center to expand the opportunities and to teach people exercises they can do at home," said Sarah.

Research studies, no matter how well designed, can't measure the contribution that nurses like Sarah Noggle make. And there are millions of them at work in hospitals, clinics, nursing homes, and village health centers around the world—nurses like Jael Waswa, who volunteers her time to offer advice and counsel at monthly HIV/AIDS meetings and at local churches in Nairobi, Kenya. "Here in Kenya nurses often have to donate their time because so many people have barely enough to pay for food on the table," she explained. And nurses like Sister Isolena and her colleagues, who run a school and clinic for the Warao Indians on Venezuela's Orinoco Delta, where tuberculosis is endemic. Their contribution to families and communities can only be hinted at in statistics. But the people they serve know full well how important they are. Accompany Jael Waswa on her visits to the teeming slums of Nairobi and you'll see smiles of gratitude on the faces of patients too sick to raise their heads. Accompany Sarah Noggle on a visit to one of her school-based clinics in Asher, Kentucky, and you'll see every child give her a hug. They all know her by name.

Nurses may begin by treating individuals, but they often end up caring for whole communities, offering not just a better chance for a healthier life but something just as precious: hope.

The pioneering work of nursing researchers around the world provides ample evidence that nursing is paramount to saving lives, lowering the risk of medical errors, and improving the quality of care and the well-being of patients. It fosters strong families, builds healthy communities, and restores human dignity and meaning to the process of dying. Short-term efforts to trim costs by cutting back nursing staffs have proved to be a dangerous failure, and not only because they put patients at risk. With health care systems in the developed world ever more burdened by rising costs, with even the most basic primary care in some of the poorest parts of the world beginning to fray, nurses often represent the slender thread that keeps health delivery from unraveling completely. Yet many nations are failing to attract, train, and support the nurses they need to meet the demand of growing populations and changing demographics.

At the same time, too many nurses, overworked and lacking the resources and support they need to do their work, are leaving the profession. The result is a crisis in nursing that both parallels and is part of the larger crisis in health care around the world—a crisis that increasingly threatens to reverse many of the advances that medicine and public health have achieved in recent years.

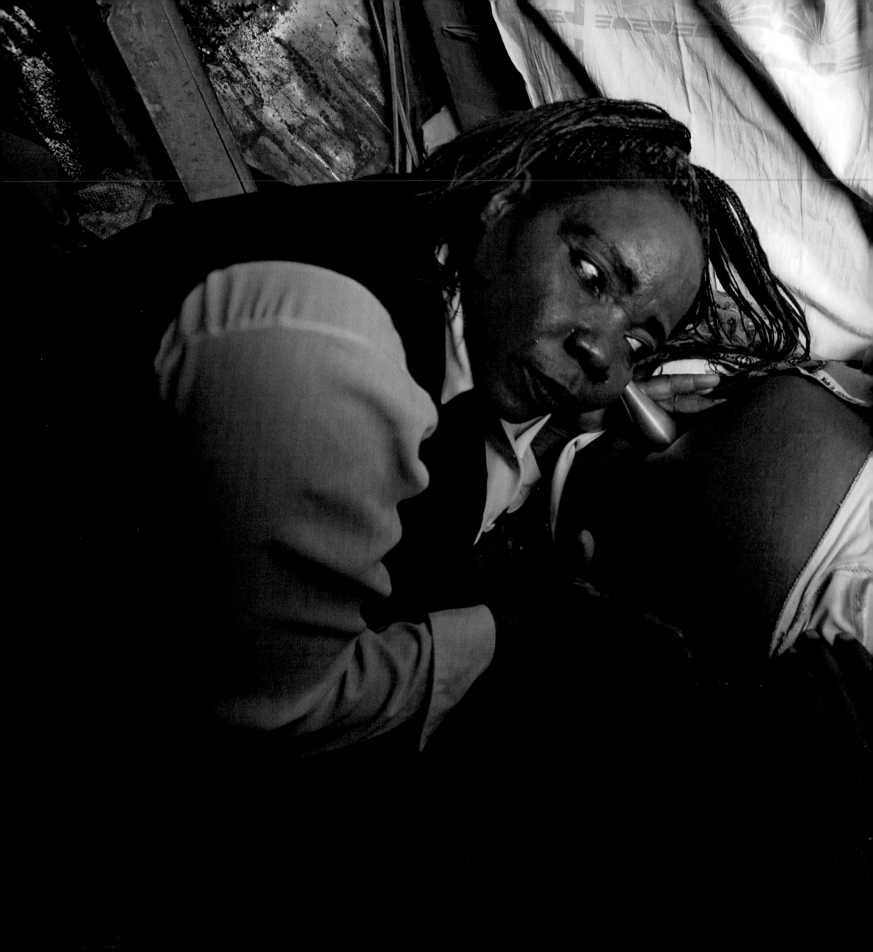

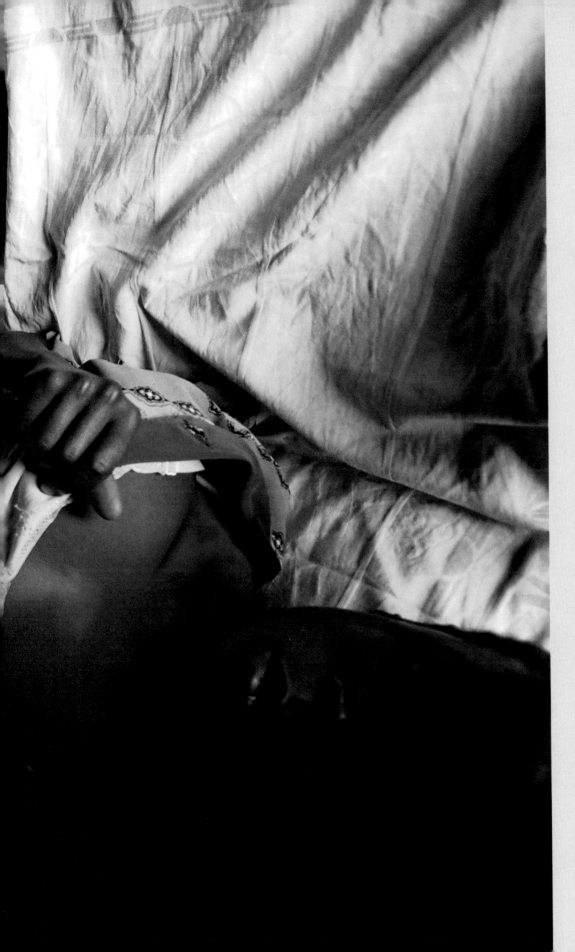

LIFE IN A NAIROBI SLUM

Kiambiu means "on the run" in Kiswahili. It's an apt name for this slum of some 30,000 people, one of the roughly 135 slum villages that have sprung up in the past decade in Nairobi, Kenya's capital. Throughout the country, people have left behind poor rural areas and migrated to the cities; most end up in over-crowded slums where water, sanitation, and schools are

Nurse and midwife Philomena Omwakwe checks on the condition of an expectant mother, one of the many impoverished residents in Nairobi's Kiambiu slum.

lacking and AIDS abundant. Nurse Philomena Omwakwe volunteers her time to help those in Kiambiu recognize and cope with the disease.

Philomena is a community outreach nurse with the Maringo Therapy Group, an off-shoot of the Friends Church. In its effort to combat AIDS, the group holds therapy support sessions for Kiambiu residents. People with AIDS who want Maringo's care must attend the sessions, designed to help destigmatize the disease and counsel those with it on ways to better control their illness through consistent medication and proper diet. The therapy sessions are also a way for nurse volunteers to hear of other people in Kiambiu who may have AIDS.

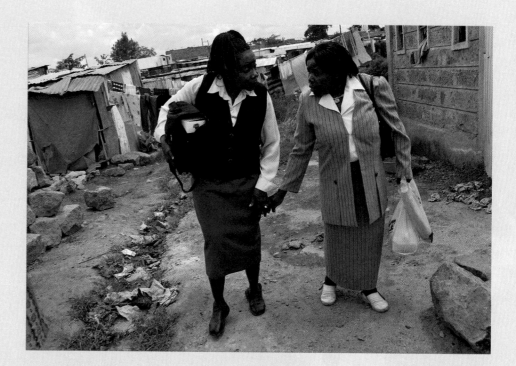

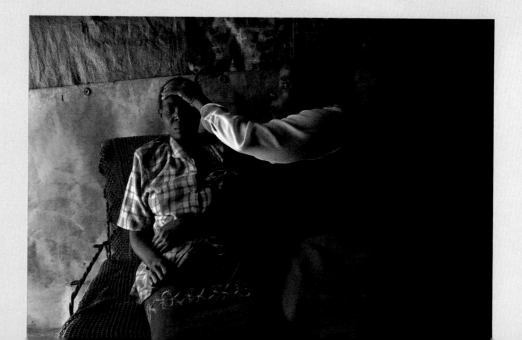

A Kiambiu mother passes on to her son the health lessons she's learned from Philomena—the importance of hand washing and wearing shoes to prevent parasitic infections. Kiambiu is a dangerous place, but Philomena (left) and her colleague Jael Waswa, on the right, stroll through it safely, because Philomena's vested uniform identifies her as a nurse—protected and respected for the care she offers residents (bottom).

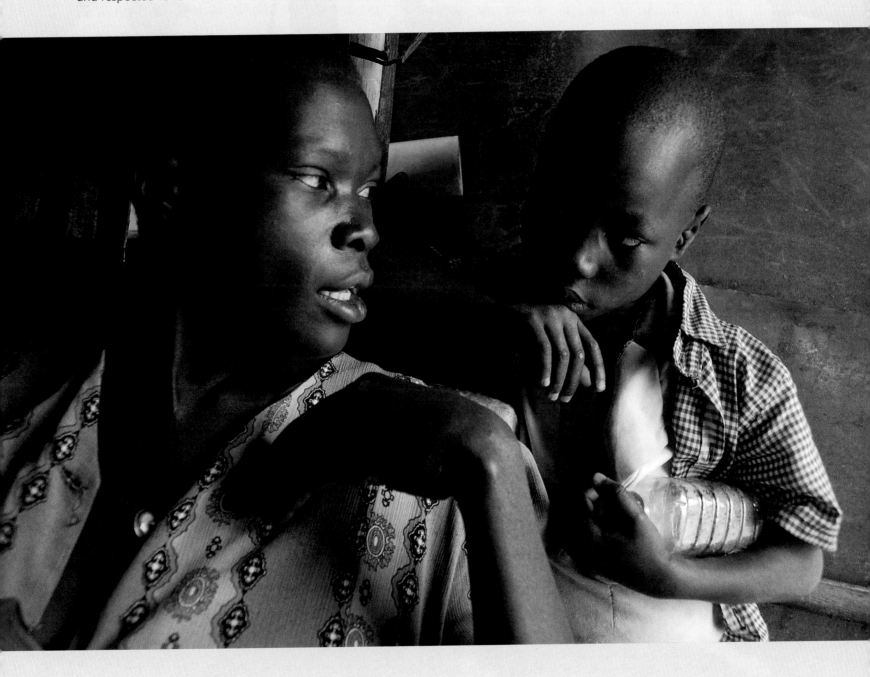

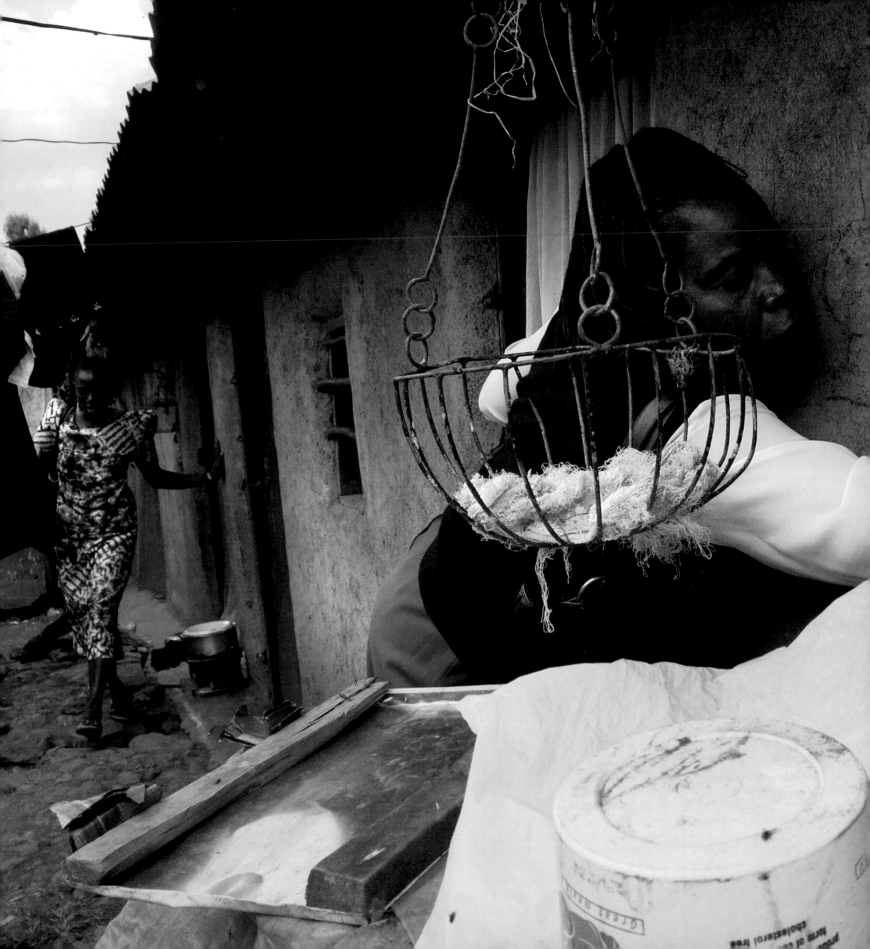

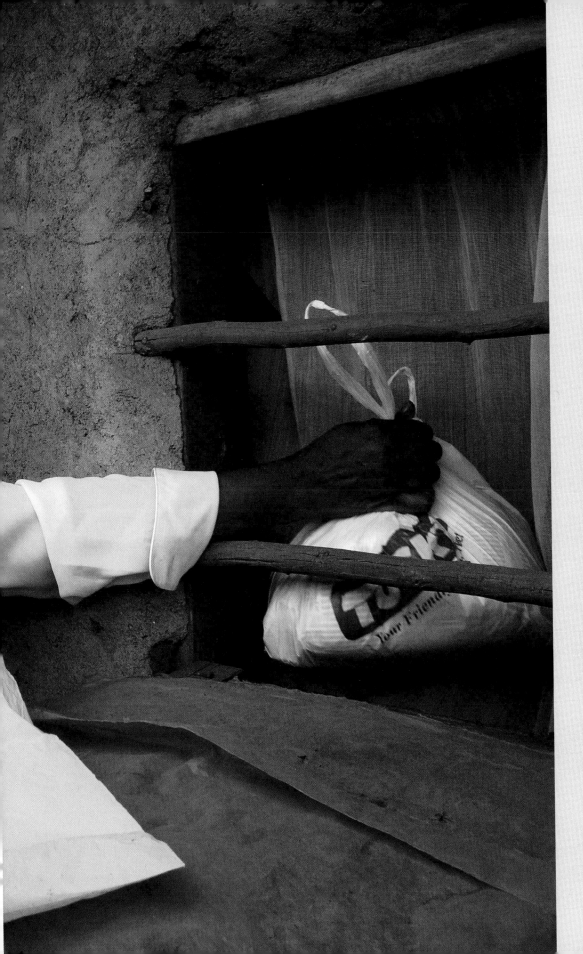

Philomena drops off a gift bag at the home of a person with AIDS. Usually donated by a foreigner visiting the Maringo Friends Church, these bags contain the simple staples of Kenyan life—corn flour, tea, sugar, and bars of soap.

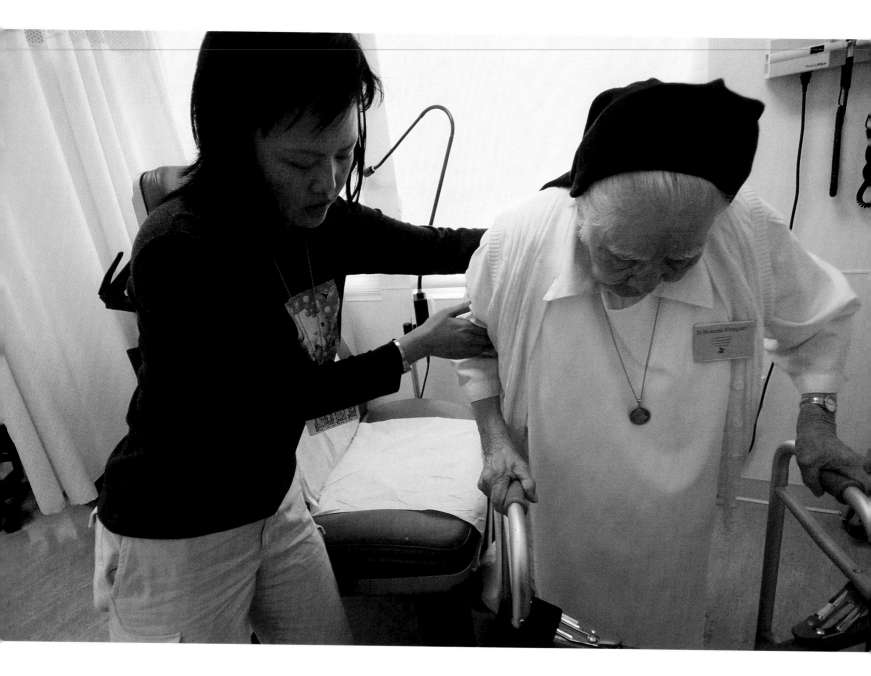

FOUR   THE LOOMING CRISIS

At a dusty rural clinic in the small African nation of Malawi, frail patients wait hours in hopes of getting access to life-saving HIV/AIDS drugs. Many will be turned away, not for lack of medicine or money but because there aren't enough nurses to meet the needs of the seemingly endless tide of sick people. As a nurse-matron working for Doctors Without Borders explained, "Our treatment program is hitting a wall because there is simply not enough nurses, doctors, and medical assistants."

In nearby Kadoma, Zimbabwe, a severe shortage of nurses endangers maternal health initiatives, AIDS treatment programs, and even campaigns to vaccinate children. The country boasted one nurse for every 700 residents in the 1990s; a decade later that ratio had fallen to one for every 7,500. Many of the country's hospitals and clinics scrape by with only 30 percent of the nurses they need for basic care.

The world's poorest countries aren't alone. In a report titled "Nursing Shortage Causes Chaos," Australia's Chief Medical Officer described patients "left in emergency department corridors for up to two days before being admitted." At least six times in a single month, all three teaching hospitals in one locale had to turn ambulances away. The reason: not enough nurses were available to receive critically ill patients.

At a senior home for Catholic sisters in San Francisco, a nurse from China offers a helping hand. Richer countries are recruiting nurses from other nations to fill shortfalls in care. But that outmigration leaves poorer countries with even fewer medical professionals.

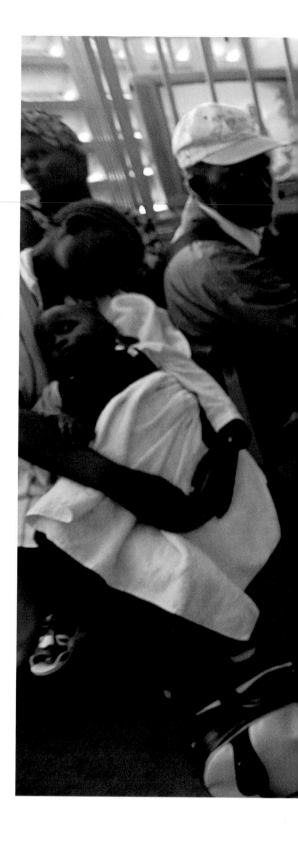

Shuttered rural clinics, understaffed hospitals, patients waiting long hours in pain or distress to be seen by a nurse—scenes like these are being repeated every day throughout the world. "I was in quite a bit of pain, but had to wait 4-6 hours to see a nurse because she was busy," one patient reported in a recent hospital survey. "Wasn't her fault, she was busy and overworked." Another described her experience as "VERY POOR. Shortage of nurses resulted in long waits for nursing attendance (bringing a bedpan). Dirty, bloody towels left in a pile on the floor. Long wait for someone to change soiled sheets."

Conditions like these might not seem surprising in an overcrowded, underfunded inner city hospital. This one happens to be a major medical facility in one of the most prosperous counties in California.

A lack of skilled nurses is nothing new. Acute nursing shortages frequently occur whenever natural disasters strike or conflicts flare. But the crisis facing health care today is different in its causes, scope, and impact. Worldwide and widening, the shortfall of nurses is seriously eroding the quality of care in many parts of the developed world, while at the same time jeopardizing efforts to improve health in poorer countries around the globe. At a time when billions of dollars from governments and charitable foundations are being directed toward improving global

Long waits greet women who come to an understaffed mother-child clinic in Houma Bay, Kenya. Nationwide, there is only one registered nurse for every 27,000 people. Many African countries have begun innovative programs to train more nurses and dissuade them from emigrating.

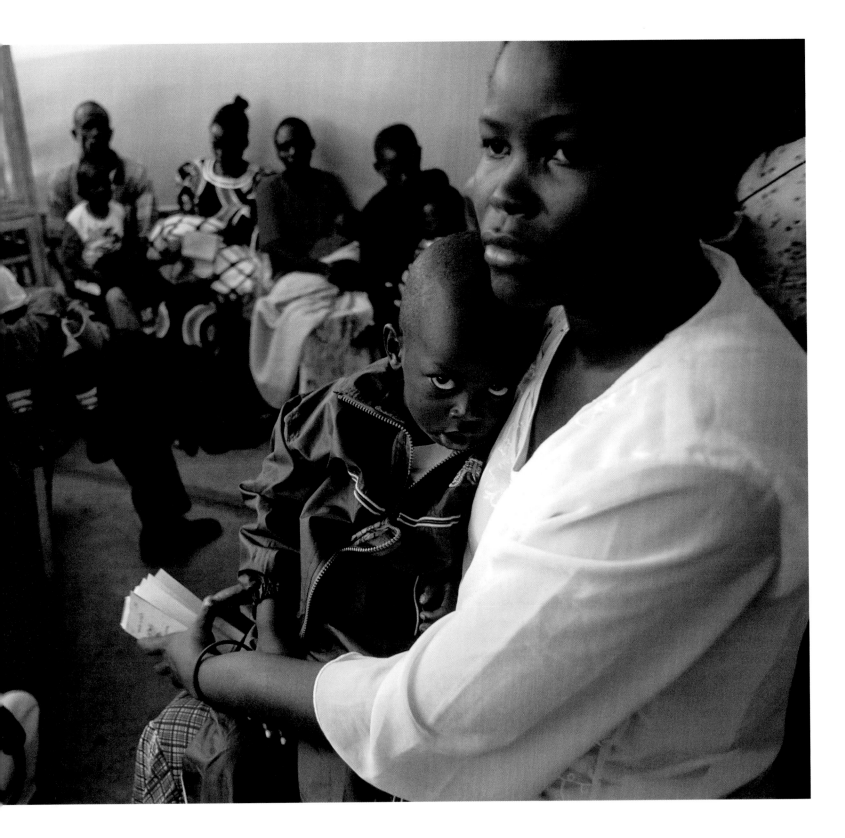

health, the lack of trained nurses has become a growing impediment to the world's best intentions. Initiatives to deliver affordable HIV/AIDS drugs have been postponed, childhood vaccine campaigns have been curtailed, and maternal health programs have been abandoned in some cases—all because there aren't enough trained nurses and other health care workers. Even where adequate numbers of trained nurses are available, the working conditions in some places have become so difficult or dangerous that a growing number of nurses are leaving the profession, just when they are needed most.

Today's crisis is being driven by a number of forces. In many resource-rich countries, the training of nurses has not kept up with increasing numbers of elderly and chronically ill people. At the same time, a growing number of nurses in the prime of their careers, discouraged by poor working conditions and the stress of having to care for more patients than they can safely manage, are leaving the profession. The resulting shortfalls have provided opportunities for nurses from poorer countries, attracting them to become part of an unprecedented global migration of nurses. This vast diaspora is made up of millions of nurses who have left homes and families to find safer and better-paying work. Jobs abroad also offer them a way to provide better lives for those left behind through the remittances they send back home.

The pull to richer countries that many nurses experience is accompanied by an equal push to leave their own because of the threat of disease, violence, and intractable poverty. As a nurse who left her husband and three children in South Africa to work in the U.K. said, "I decided with my husband that I should come over. It's not nice leaving your family,

The shortfall of nurses is seriously eroding the quality of care in many parts of the developed world, while at the same time jeopardizing efforts to improve health in poorer countries.

leaving your country. I didn't do it deliberately, I was pushed." Indeed, poor and sometimes dangerous working conditions, low wages, stress, and the overwhelming burdens created by the HIV/AIDS epidemic are compelling a growing number of nurses to leave South Africa, an exodus that jeopardizes even basic health care delivery. As a director of nursing in that country put it, "We are at a level of desperation."

In the Republic of Mauritius, on the east coast of Africa, the flight of nurses happened so quickly that health officials were caught almost completely by surprise. "In just three years, between 2003 and 2005, we lost over 800 qualified nurses, or about 25 percent of our workforce," said Francis Supparayen, coordinator of international nursing affairs for Mauritius. "Worst of all for us, the nurses who were leaving were the ones with specialized skills, the ones who worked in intensive care units, cardiac centers, operating theaters—the ones who are caring for the sickest, most vulnerable patients. And the ones who are most difficult for us to replace."

The small island nation isn't alone. More than 500 nurses left the African nation of Ghana in 2000, twice the number of new nurses graduating that year. In 2003, a single hospital in Swaziland lost one in three of its nurses for work abroad. By 2005, Botswana was losing 60 percent of its newly trained health care workers annually to emigration.

The flight has decimated health care in many of the poorest corners of the world. In an influential report published in 2006, the World Health Organization identified 57 countries that face critical shortages of health care workers, including doctors, nurses, and trained midwives. The most severe shortages are found in countries in Africa and Southeast Asia.

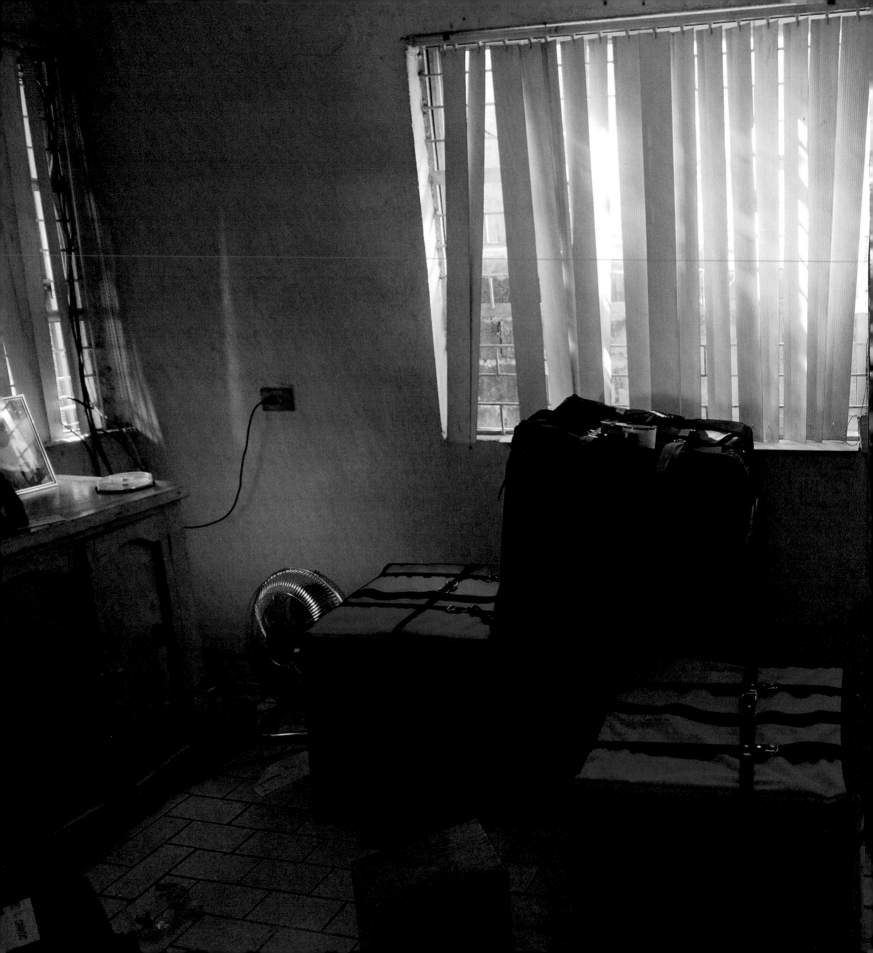

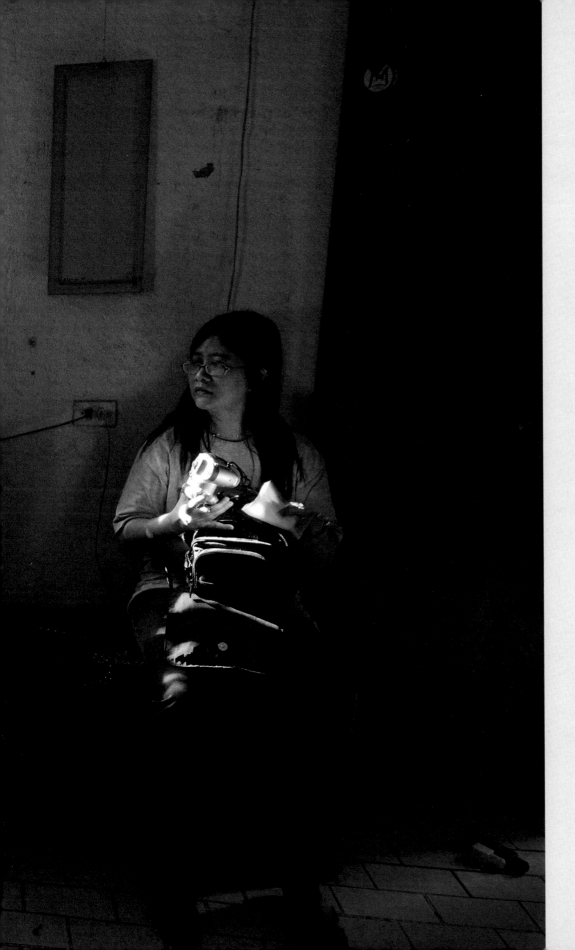

EXPORTING NURSES

You could say Patricia Gamacho is one of the lucky ones. Recruited by a senior-care facility in California, she's among the many Filipina nurses who outmigrate annually. But she has managed to get visas for her husband and three children to come with her, even though it took two years to do so. That's good for the Gamacho family, but it's not so good for the Philippines, which is losing both a nurse and a qualified nursing instructor.

Packed and pensive, Filipina nurse Patricia Gamacho contemplates her move across the planet to a new life in California.

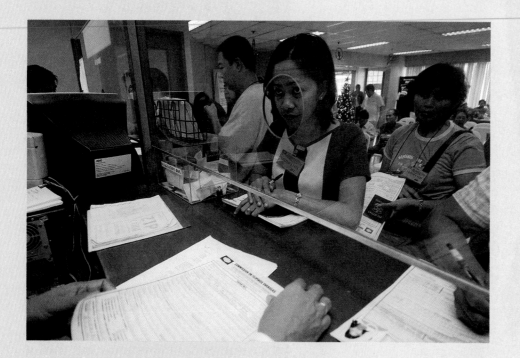

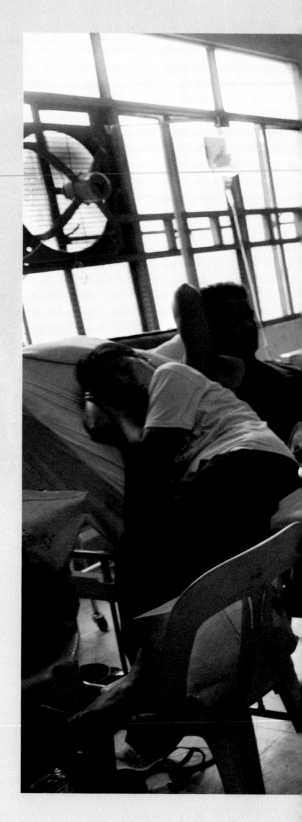

At a crowded hospital in Manila (right), families wait in the emergency room's overflow area, where a student nurse is assigned to evaluate their conditions. Above: Anxiously awaiting approval to immigrate to California, a Filipina nurse presents her visa papers to the Commission on Filipinos Overseas.

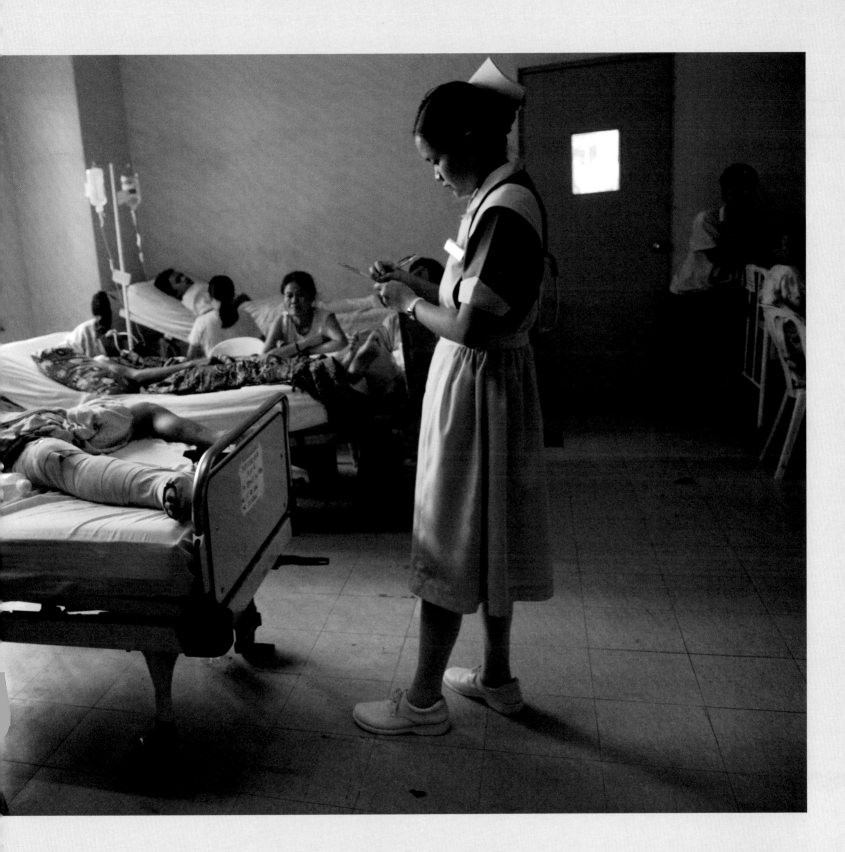

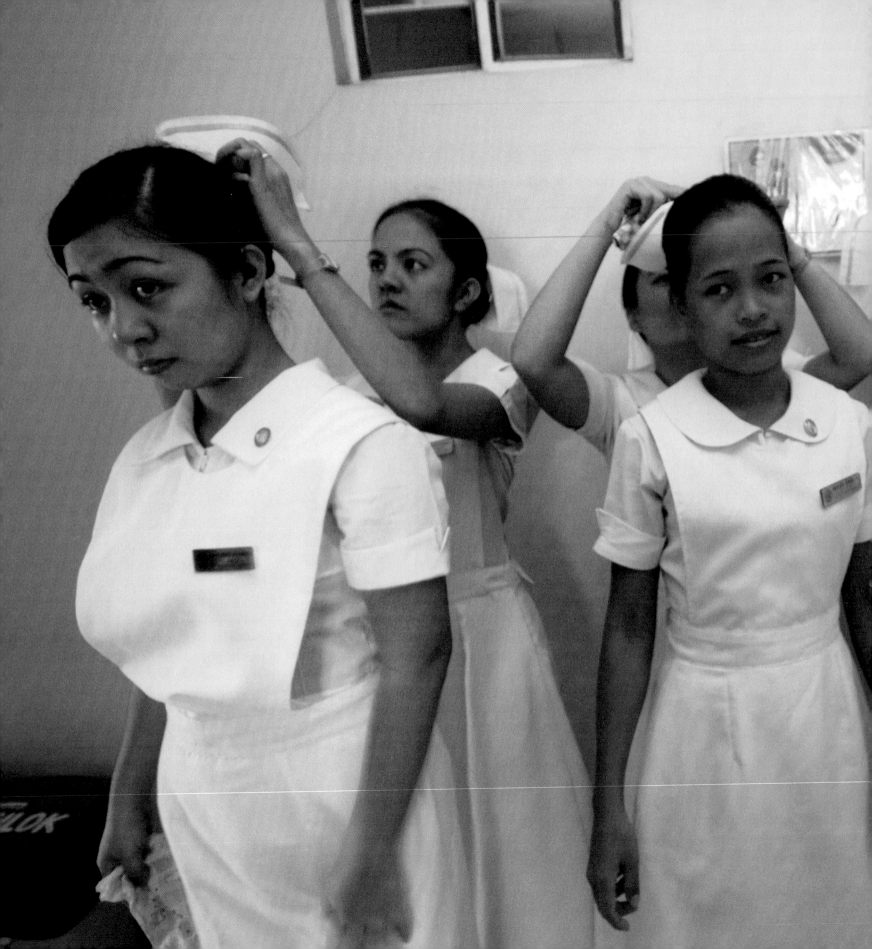

The Philippine government has long encouraged emigration among its skilled professionals. The incentive for outmigration is usually simple economics: The average nursing salary in the Philippines is some 40 percent lower than that of a nurse's aide in the U.S. The desire for a better life is driving roughly 10,000 Filipino nurses and doctors to emigrate annually. Yet outmigration also leads to "de-skilling"— that is, imported nurses and doctors are often given lesser jobs in their new countries— and the Philippines itself is left "de-skilled," with fewer medical personnel to deal with its citizens' health needs.

At Batangas Regional Hospital, nursing students ready one another for a day on the floor. Many Manila hospitals have so many nursing students that there aren't enough trained nurses to supervisor them properly.

Sub-Saharan Africa, for instance, has 11 percent of the world's population, 24 percent of the disease burden—yet barely 3 percent of the world's health workers. In some African hospitals, a single nurse may be responsible for 50 patients, far more than even the most dedicated professional can manage. Haiti, which has seen the loss of many of its health professionals, has barely one nurse per 10,000 inhabitants.

In the Philippines, nurses have become one of the country's leading exports. Over 70 percent of nurse graduates leave the country to work abroad each year. Some 164,000 Filipino nurses—85 percent of the country's trained total—work outside the country. At José Reyes Memorial Hospital in Manila, which operates its own nurse training program, as many as nine out of ten of the newly trained nurses will be gone within six months, leaving for countries with higher-paying jobs. Small wonder. Nurses working in a Philippine hospital can expect to make about $100 a month. In the U.S. or Japan, they can earn $4,000 or more.

THE MOBILITY OF TODAY'S GLOBAL NURSING WORKFORCE HAS ITS BENEFITS. Nurses working abroad can send money home, putting food on the family's table and giving their children an education. These remittances represent an important source of revenue in countries like the Philippines or Zambia. They help to redress, at least partially, the global inequity in wealth that spurs migration in the first place.

And there are other benefits. Many nurses go abroad to take advantage of educational and training opportunities. "The global movement of nurses has opened up opportunities that simply don't exist for many nurses at home," said Mireille Kingma, an expert on migration at the

Like so many nurses, Boaz Sikobe saw a need and addressed it. Sikobe works in a private children's clinic in Nairobi but volunteers here at the Mama Ngina Kenyatta Children's Home, where he originally expected to assist with a CDC-sponsored safe-water project. But when he realized that many babies coming to the orphanage received no medical evaluation, he began giving them check-ups himself.

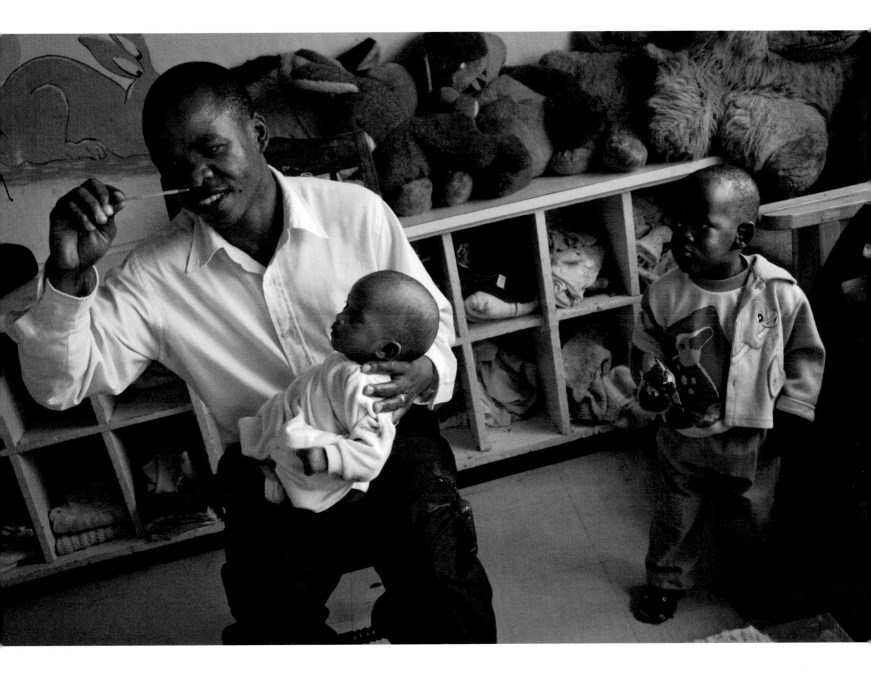

International Council of Nursing and the author of *Nurses on the Move: Migration and the Global Health Care Economy*. "Under the best circumstances, nurses return home with new skills, new experience, new training. In that case, migration represents a valuable brain exchange, rather than a brain drain."

But in reality, most nurses don't return—and their departures have left not only primary health care but also nurse training programs in many of the world's poorer countries in tatters. As a director of nursing in the Philippines said, "I am left with only novice nurses . . . . Our experienced ones go . . . who will teach the novice nurse?"

In 1995, the General Agreement on Trade in Services directly addressed the issue of the movement of nurses and other health professionals across borders. Because of the severe dislocations that have occurred, some policy makers urged countries that import nurses to reciprocate by supporting efforts to expand nursing education in the countries they tap. So far those calls haven't gained much traction. Nor have governments or private aid organizations placed enough emphasis on training to counterbalance the loss of nursing resources. And many experts worry that there are inherent dangers in treating nurses as a commodity to be traded in the global marketplace. If finance ministers negotiate trade agreements for nurses without the involvement of ministers of health, for example, the national treasury may benefit at the expense of health care delivery on the ground. The problem is exacerbated by the rise of so-called health tourism. In countries like Thailand and India, a growing number of hospitals and clinics offer foreigners discounted health care procedures such as heart surgery, knee replacements, dental implants,

> "Under the best circumstances, nurses [who emigrate] return home with new skills, new experience, new training. In that case, migration represents a valuable brain exchange, rather than a brain drain."
>
> *Mireille Kingma*

and even facelifts, putting additional strain on already threadbare local health resources.

Migration across borders is only part of the problem. A vast movement of nurses and other health care workers is also taking place within national boundaries, as more and more skilled and educated people are leaving the countryside for the city. Today, 75 percent of doctors and 60 percent of nurses reside in urban areas, according to the WHO, compared to just 55 percent of the general population. That leaves many rural areas with virtually no health care at all.

Ironically, the work of international aid organizations is inadvertently fueling some of the imbalances in the distribution of health resources around the world. Huge amounts of money are pouring into global health initiatives. That's welcome news, of course. But well-funded international health or relief organizations can often offer nurses and doctors far more than can the Ministry of Health or local hospitals. As a result, high-profile programs such as HIV/AIDS drug delivery or polio vaccination campaigns may have plenty of staff, while programs to fight childhood dysentery or other lower-profile diseases go begging. In the worst cases, already strained basic primary health care delivery systems are being torn asunder. As Laurie Garrett, senior fellow for global health at the Council on Foreign Relations, wrote in a recent issue of the journal *Foreign Affairs*, "Even as money has poured into Ghana for HIV/AIDS and malaria programs, the country has moved backward on other health markers. Prenatal care, maternal health programs, the treatment of guinea worm, measles vaccination efforts—all have declined as the country has shifted its health-care workers to the better-funded projects."

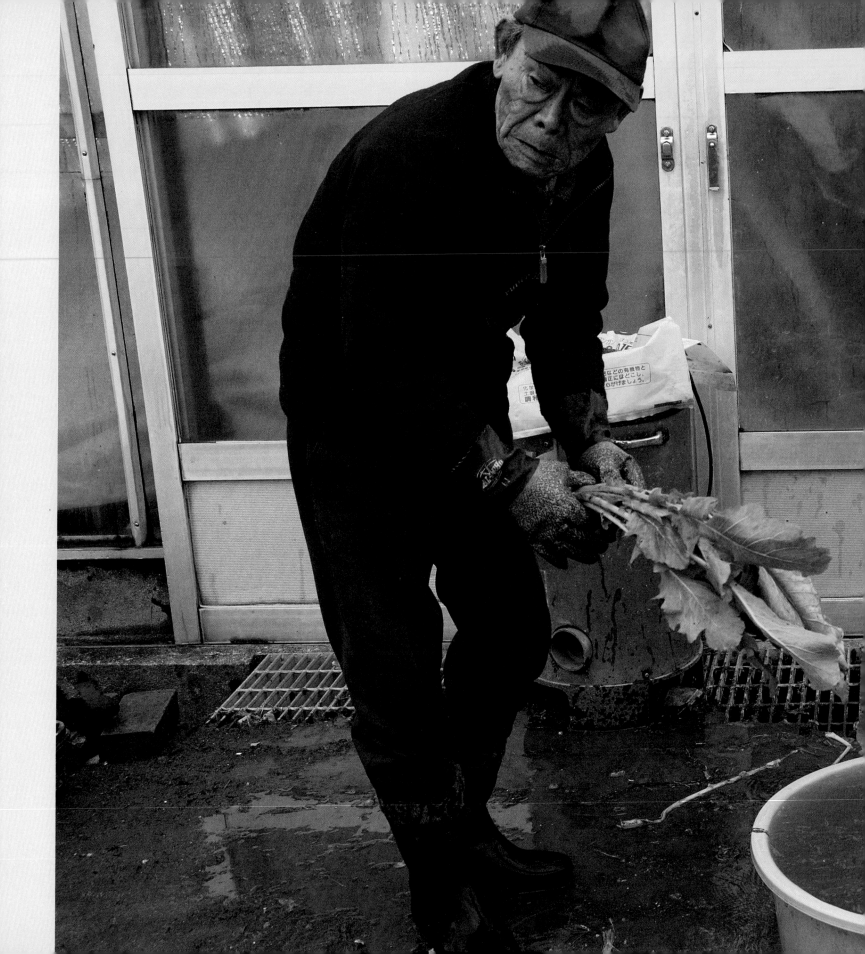

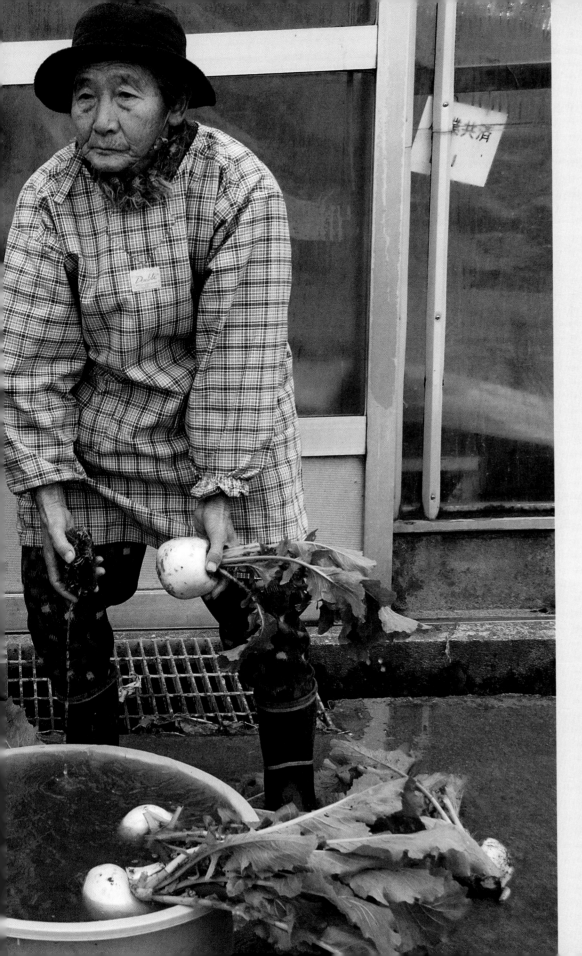

AGING IN JAPAN

Growing old in Japan has never held the stigma that it presents in many Western nations. Respected in Japan, the elderly were traditionally cared for by their families, usually the women members, in their homes. Now, things are shifting, as Japan faces a demographic tipping point, with those over 65 accounting for roughly 20 percent of the population. Government and private industry "silver businesses" have risen to the challenge, with a variety of options

In their 80s, the Hashizumes still grow vegetables on their small farm in Nanto City, but much of Japan's burgeoning elderly population now needs some kind of daily assistance.

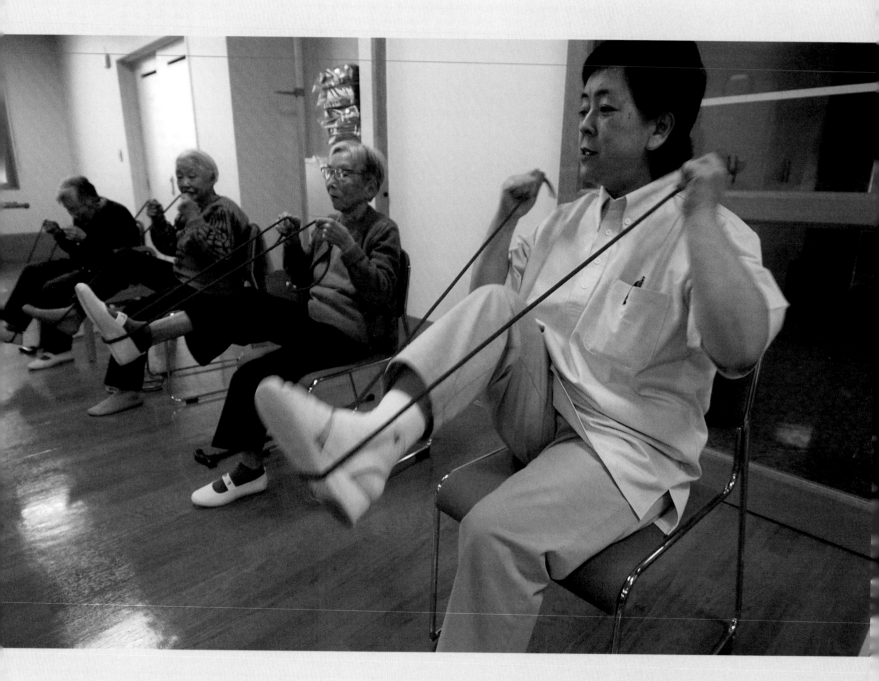

At the Inami Dayservice Center in Nanto City, nurses work hard to keep participants active with exercises, entertainment, and interaction with a robotic seal that responds to their touch with movement and mewing.

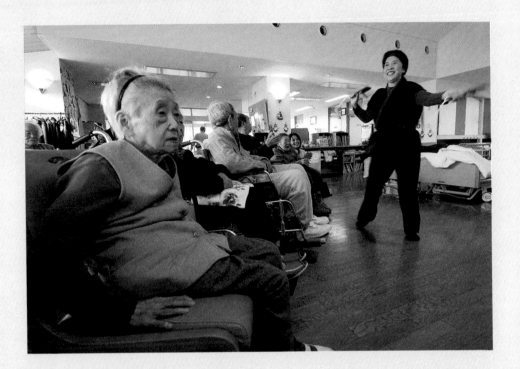

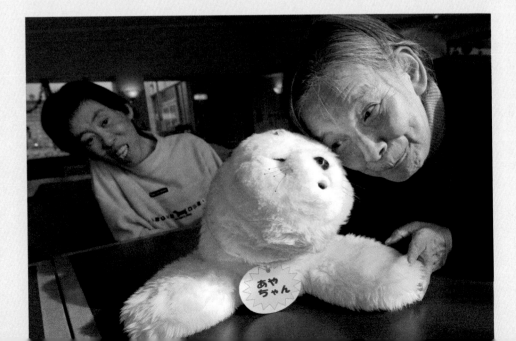

for aging citizens and their families. Nurses caring for the elderly are well trained and well paid.

Robots, bathing services, even services that take the elderly on vacation are on the rise in Japan, all aimed at older people coping on their own. As social mores have changed and the population has become more mobile, many aging Japanese now live alone. A number of daycare centers, run by private and government organizations, offer the elderly stimulation and companionship. With the average life expectancy among Japanese men hovering at 79 and women at 86, the country has among the highest longevity rates in the world—and a live birthrate in decline. For almost two decades, the government has been carefully planning ways to ensure a good quality of life for its older citizens.

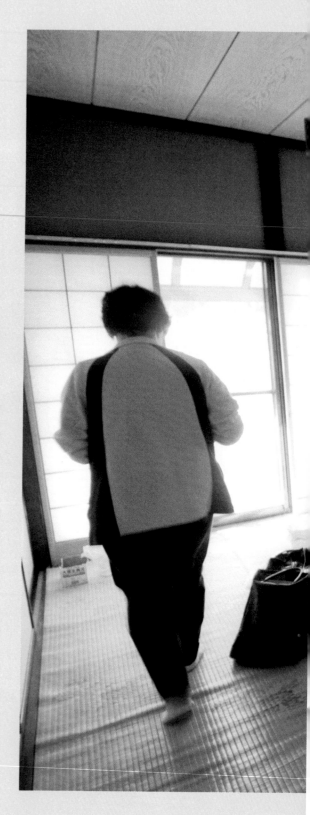

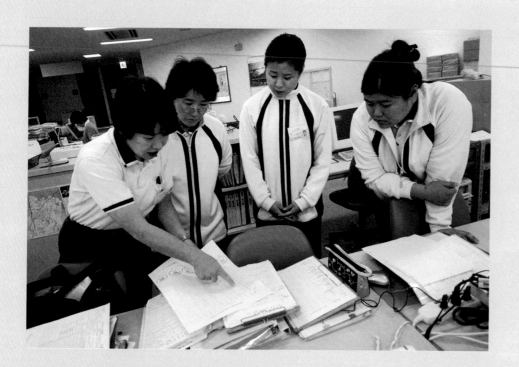

A team of home-visit nurses, employees of the Nanto City government, meets to plan the day's agenda. Each will check on the health of elderly patients. Outside the bedroom of a woman close to death, her son (right) waits patiently, as the home-health nurse makes her visit. The nurses are on 24-hour call, should emergencies arise.

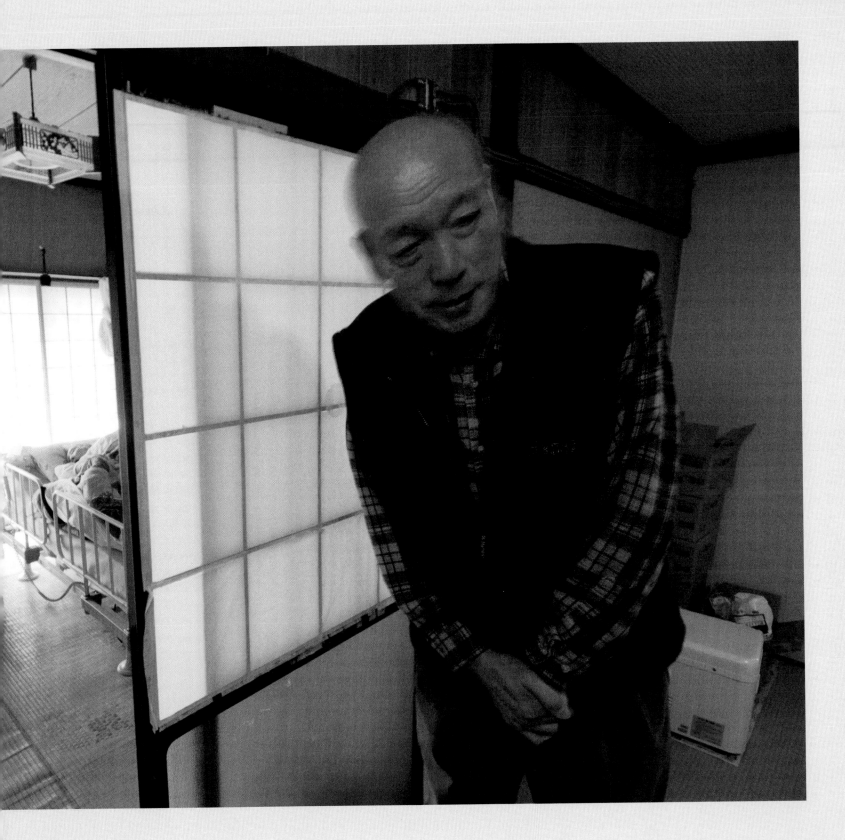

THE WORLD'S PROSPEROUS COUNTRIES REMAIN THE MOST POWERFUL MAGNETS for nurses from the developing world. Many, in fact, have been aggressively recruiting nurses from the poorest corners of the world, including Africa, Southeast Asia, and the Philippines. One in five nurses now working in New Zealand was trained abroad. One in three nurses in Switzerland is foreign educated. More than 8 percent of registered nurses working in the U.S. were educated abroad. Among them, well over 80,000 came from the Philippines. Another 47,000 emigrated from the Caribbean and Latin America. Although the U.S. now imports more nurses than any other country in the world, the U.K. until recently wasn't far behind. In 2002, the number of foreign-educated nurses entering the workforce there exceeded the number of newly qualified nurses educated in the U.K.

Countries around the world have opened their doors to nurses for a simple reason. As the need for skilled nursing care has climbed, many of the world's most prosperous countries have failed to attract, train, and retain enough nurses on their own. The dramatic expansion in medical therapies has dramatically increased the demand for nurses. So have growing populations and especially the soaring number of elderly people. Most countries simply aren't keeping up. In the U.S. today, some 85 percent of hospitals are currently having trouble hiring nurses to fill vacant positions. By 2020, according to estimates by the Health Resources and Service Administration, the nation could face a shortage of a million nurses. According to the WHO, a staggering 4.3 million nurses, midwives, and doctors are needed worldwide to meet current demand. Many more will be needed in the future.

The shortfall has created conditions in which patients are often in

Nursing has failed to attract significant numbers of men to the profession. By the latest estimate only 6 percent of registered nurses in the U.S. are male.

real danger. In a survey published in 2002 in the *New England Journal of Medicine*, 53 percent of doctors and 65 percent of the public cited the shortage of nurses as the leading cause of medical errors. Several years ago, the Joint Commission on Accreditation of Healthcare Organizations examined 1,609 hospital records of patient deaths and injuries. Inadequate nursing staff levels, the report concluded, were a factor in 24 percent of the incidents.

Why are nurses in such short supply, even in prosperous countries? Social changes are partly to blame. The job of attracting and training nurses faces several challenges. Nursing has historically been able to attract large numbers of women because it was one of the most welcoming professional careers available to them; today, many more career paths are available, some potentially far more lucrative than nursing. At the same time, even as more and more occupations are shared equally by men and women, nursing has failed to attract significant numbers of men to the profession. By the latest estimate only 6 percent of registered nurses in the U.S. are male. And though the overall number of registered nurses is growing in the U.S, it isn't enough to meet the demands of growing populations and aging demographics.

To be sure, there are encouraging signs of a resurgence of interest in the profession of nursing among young people. By putting global health in the spotlight, organizations like the Carter Center and the Bill & Melinda Gates Foundation have inspired more and more people to consider careers in public health nursing. Unfortunately, many won't be able to pursue that dream. Even as hospitals scramble to fill vacant nursing positions and many health clinics struggle to maintain adequate nursing staff levels, nursing schools are turning away qualified applicants. In the U.S., for example, an estimated 41,683 applicants were unable to find a place in the country's baccalaureate and graduate nursing programs in 2005—not because they weren't qualified but because of a combination of faculty shortages, lack of clinical and classroom space, and budget constraints. Three out of four nursing schools say faculty shortages are the main reason they have to turn away qualified entry-level nurses.

At the same time, many trained nurses in the U.S. and other countries are leaving the profession before they reach retirement age. In a survey published in *Health Affairs* in 2001, researchers found two out of five nurses working in hospitals were dissatisfied with their jobs. One in three under the age of 30 planned to leave those jobs within the next year. Nurses represent a precious resource. Yet according to one recent survey, fewer than six in ten registered nurses worked full-time, 25 percent worked part-time, and 16.8 percent—more than one in six—were no longer employed in nursing. By 2005, roughly half a million registered nurses had given up working in the profession.

There are many reasons why nurses choose to leave the profession, of course, from the demands of raising a family to the attraction of other career opportunities. Unfortunately, many nurses are calling it quits simply because they're burning out. The burnout rate among nurses is as high as 43 percent, among the highest for any profession. Nursing has always been stressful, of course. People's health, after all, and often their lives, are in the hands of nurses. Most nurses love the challenge. But with nursing staffs overstretched, with hospitals and other institutions cutting back on the resources that support nursing, with the strains of

Duck farms have always been part of the landscape in Thailand, but with the threat of avian influenza, the farms have become potential breeding grounds for more than poultry. Thanks to a CDC-sponsored surveillance program aimed at respiratory diseases and coordinated by research nurses in the field, farmers have been given guidelines to help reduce the risk of the deadly influenza.

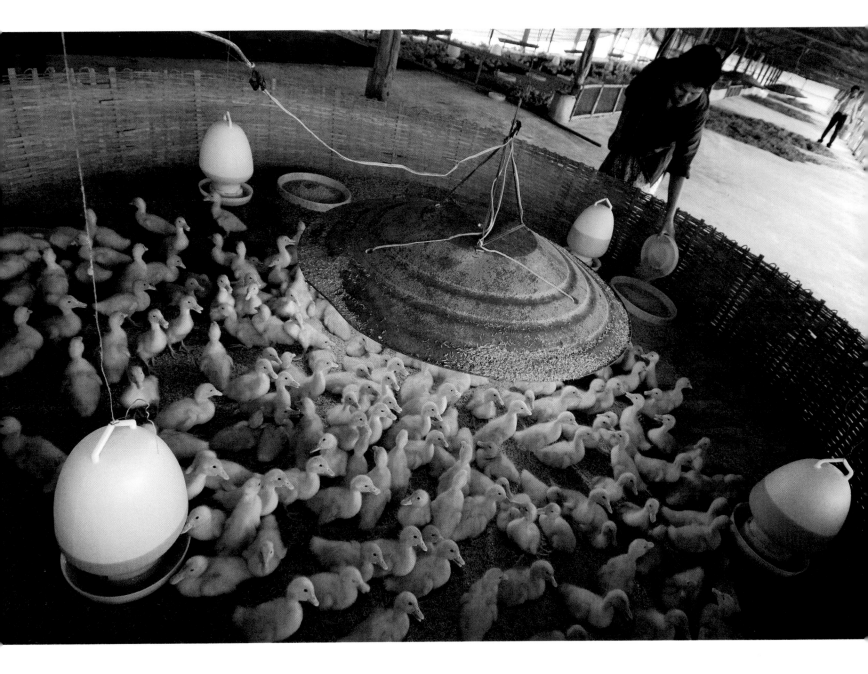

A land of refugees, the Meuy River corridor separates Thailand from Burma, where persecution of ethnic minorities has led many to flee across the border. This health aid worker, a refugee herself, is gathering water from the only source available—the river. War, persecution, famine, and drought have left an estimated 33 million people worldwide displaced from their homes and often without access to health care.

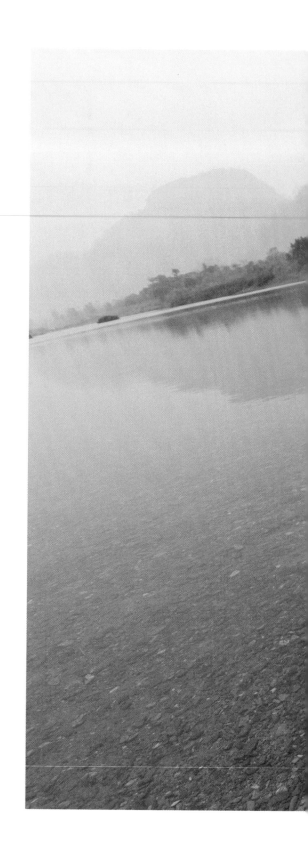

the larger health care crisis beginning to tear at the fabric of the relationship between patients and health care providers, more and more nurses say they can no longer do the work of caring that attracted them to the profession in the first place.

Ray Bingham is one of them. A registered nurse certified in neonatal intensive care, he gave up working at the bedside in 1995--and later wrote movingly of his reasons in the journal *Health Affairs*. Bingham was a specialist in a technology that keeps the most desperately fragile premature babies alive, called extracorporeal membrane oxygenation, or ECMO. His moment of disillusionment came on a day when, after repeated cutbacks, his neonatal unit was dangerously understaffed. Bingham voiced his concerns. Hospital administrators ignored him. He went back to work. "But something inside me was missing; something had flamed out," he wrote. Later, one of the premature babies in the unit developed a severe intestinal infection that could have been avoided with adequate vigilance. Another died because, in Bingham's view, there weren't enough trained nurses on duty. Eventually, he left nursing at the bedside. "I still feel about nursing as I always have," he wrote, "that it is an honorable and noble profession, affecting countless lives by providing a caring, honest, human touch in times of great distress. I love nursing. I just can't do it anymore."

LIKE BINGHAM, MOST NURSES LOVE WHAT THEY DO. THAT SIMPLE YET powerful fact holds out a beacon of hope in the face of the current crisis in nursing and in health care in general. In a recent poll of nurses in ten countries conducted by the International Council of Nurses, respondents

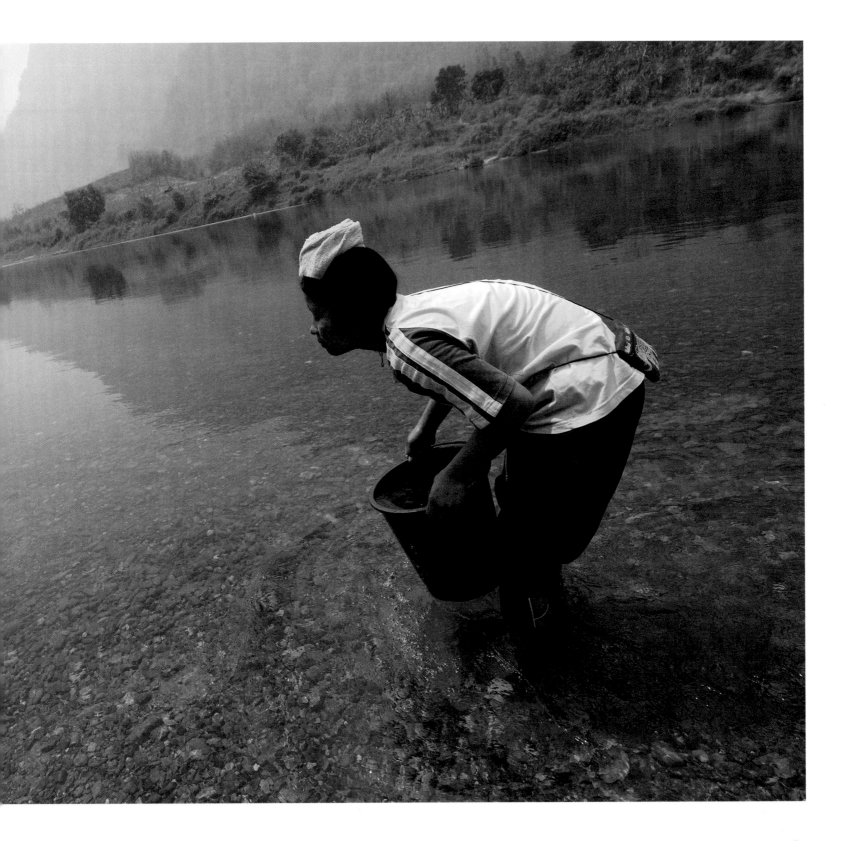

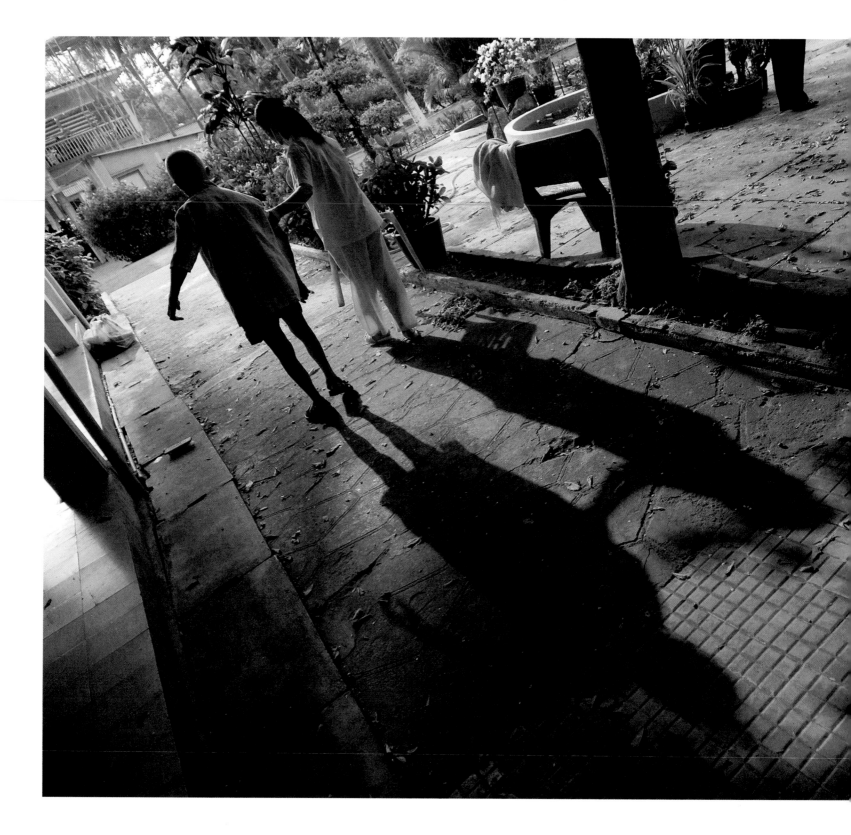

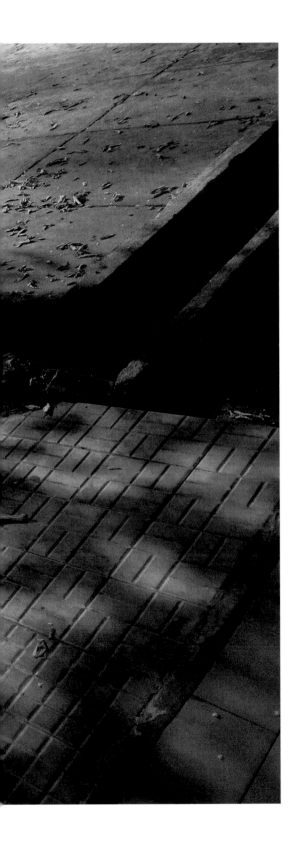

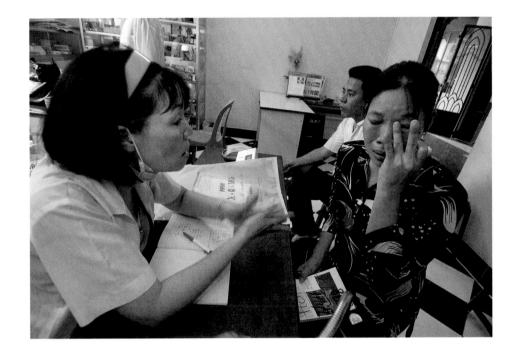

Shadows of a long-dreaded disease follow residents at the Ben San Leprosy Treatment Center (left) in Ho Chi Minh City. Many of the nurses here first came to the center with loved ones who were leprosy patients; they learned nursing skills then stayed on to help others. Those suspecting that they have the newest dread disease in Vietnam and much of Southeast Asia—HIV/AIDS—can go to the Catholic-supported Phu Trung Clinic (above), also in Ho Chi Minh City, where they receive testing and, if necessary, treatment. The woman on the right has just received news that her results were positive.

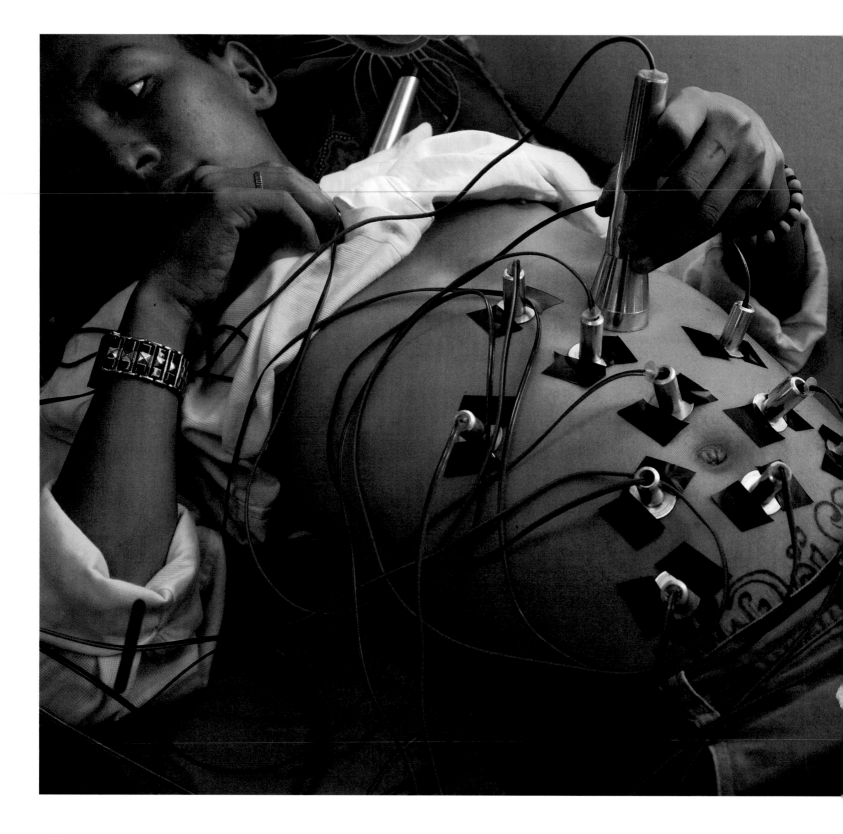

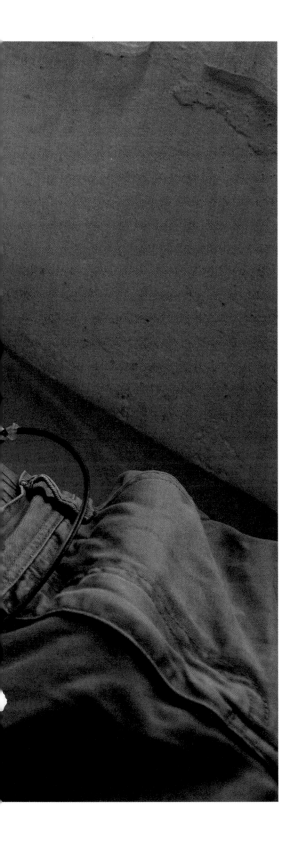

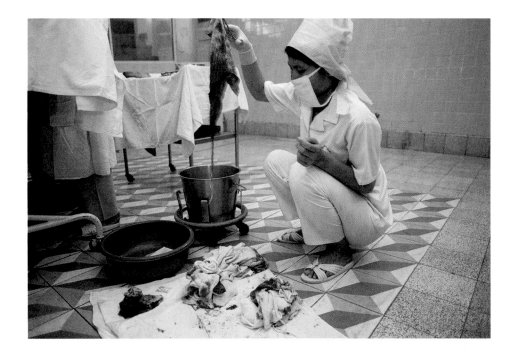

Combining traditional acupuncture with laser technology (left),
the Mai Khoi Clinic in Saigon offers AIDS patients a new way of deal-
ing with the disease. Such high-tech tools are a far cry from former
conditions in Vietnamese hospitals, where bloody towels were washed
by hand for reuse (above).

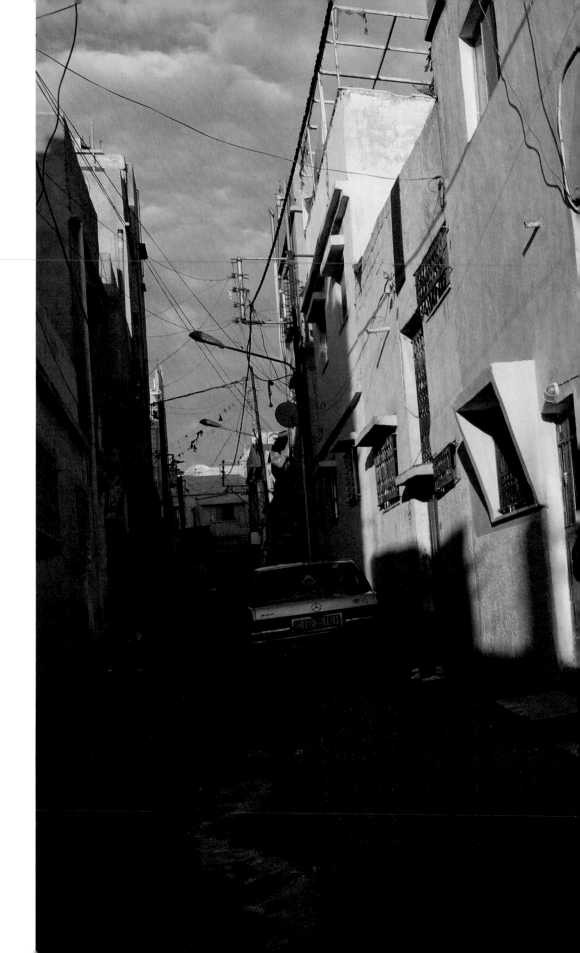

Aspiring to a better life, Khulood, a young Palestinian woman in a refugee community in Amman, Jordan, is pursuing a degree in nursing. Her income as a nurse will likely provide much of the financial support for her family.

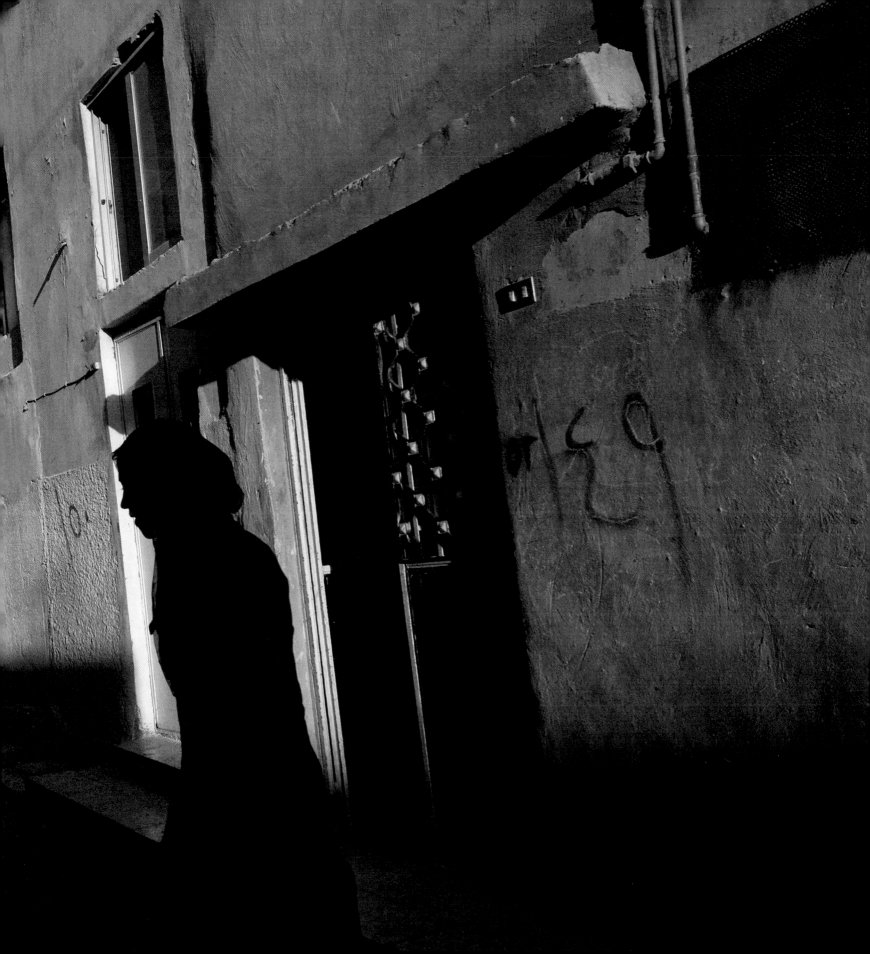

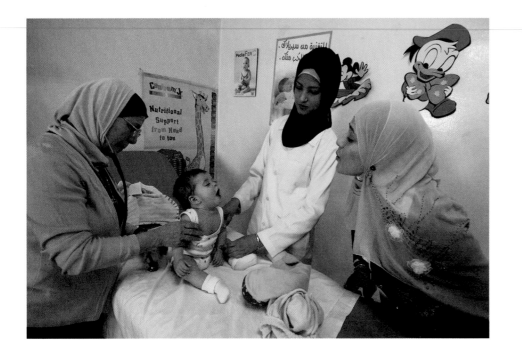

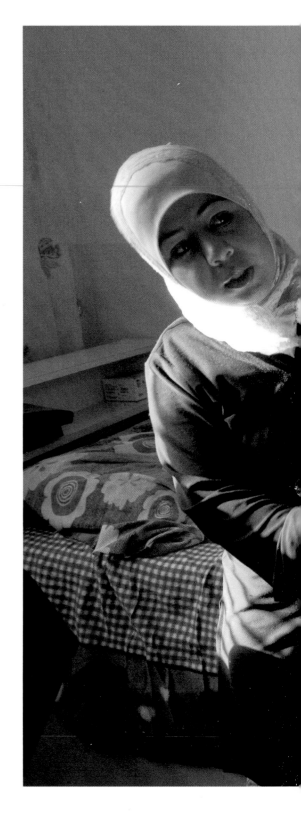

Watching and learning led Dalal, (right, in a headscarf) to nursing.
When her sister, middle, was hospitalized with a genetic disorder, Dalal
paid close attention to the nursing care and decided to become a nurse.
Jordanian secondary schools offer basic training as a nurse. Further
college training is an unaffordable luxury for most Palestinian refugees,
but Khulood (above, in a black headscarf) is being sponsored by Dr. Hanan,
at left, a pediatrician who maintains the clinic where Khulood works.

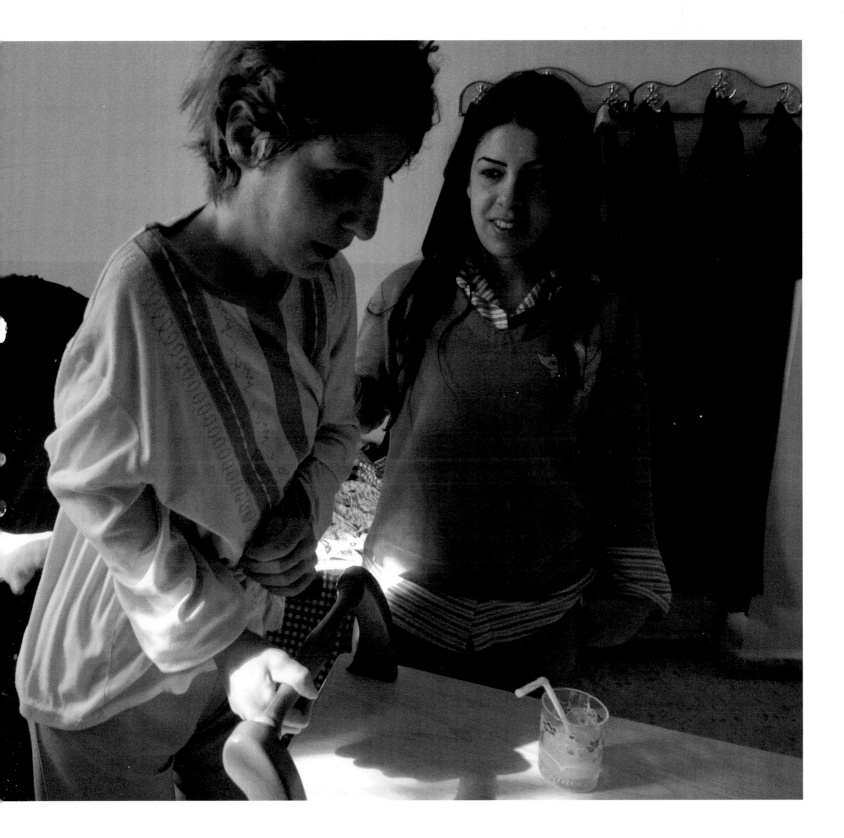

frequently complained about having too little time to care for patients, too much work, low salaries, and poor working conditions. But they still placed high value on the profession and the work of nursing. "The findings tell us that nurses everywhere are upbeat about their work as professional and compassionate health care providers," Hiroko Minami, president of ICN, said. "At the same time they say health care systems need to do a better job at creating environments where nurses and all health professionals are enabled to do well what they do best—provide quality care to patients."

That's already happening. Around the world, nurses are speaking out about the challenges they face. Just as important, they are offering ingenious solutions that will allow them to better care for patients. Governments and international aid organizations are beginning to recognize the crucial role that nurses can make in improving the quality of care and access to it. Policy makers are taking note. Indeed, the current crisis in nursing has etched in bold relief the contribution that nursing can make to solving many of the problems we face, not only in providing health care but in creating the conditions that will give people everywhere a fair chance at living a healthy life.

School books in hand, Khulood faces a future far brighter than many Palestinian refugees. Once she's completed her nursing education, she will be in great demand. The 13 Palestinian refugee camp-communities scattered across Jordan are home to 1.6 million people, but the doctors and nurses to serve them are in short supply; many of the best educated nurses leave the camps for better-paying jobs with the UN or with nongovernmental organizations.

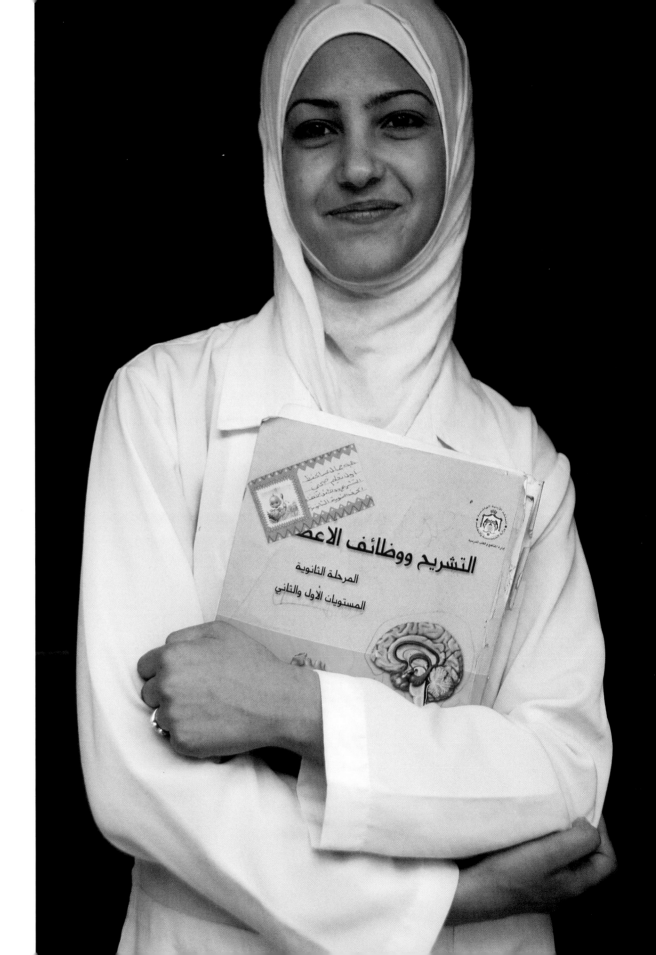

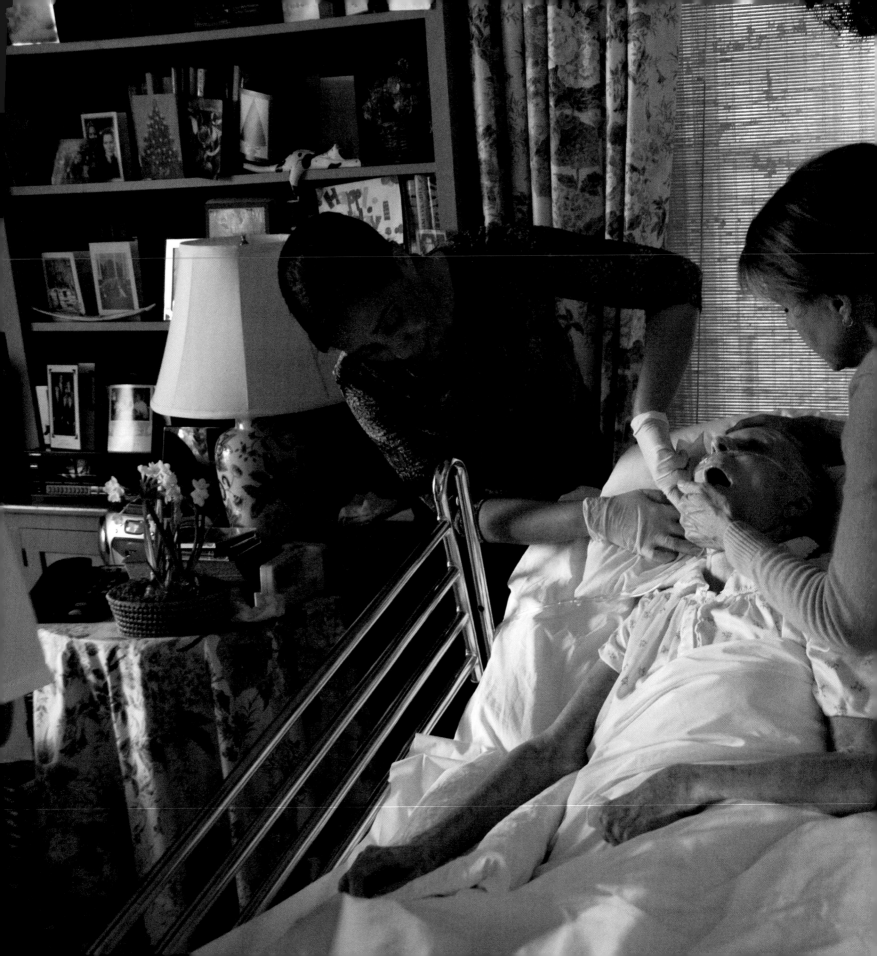

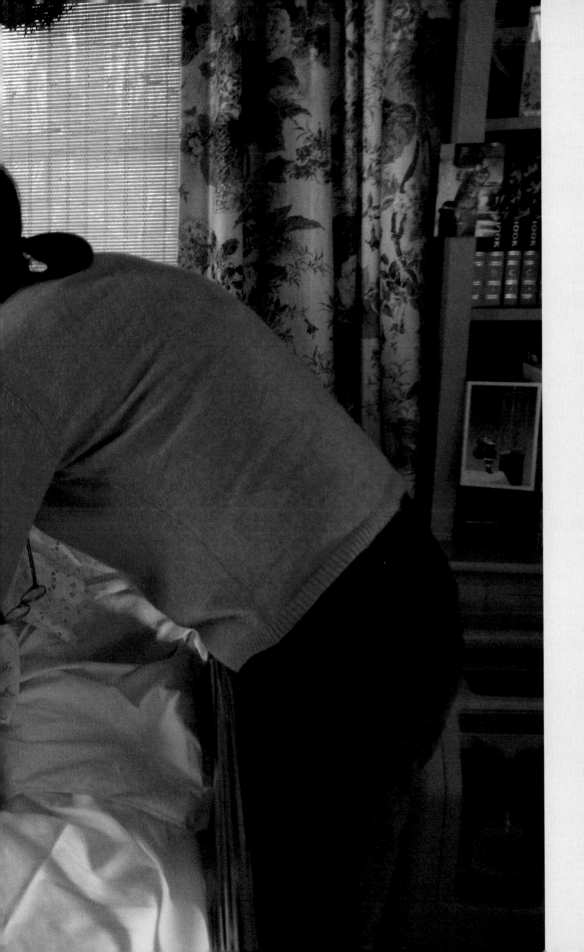

A KINDER PASSING

Nurses are there when we come into the world, and they're there again to help us leave it gently. In recent decades, nursing has become the vital component in ever-expanding hospice care. With nurses by the bedside of the dying, offering the palliative care needed to ease pain, the final days of life can be spent at home, comforted by familiar surroundings and the intimacy of family and friends.

As the end approaches, Mrs. Elene Gill is cared for in her Washington, D.C., home by hospice nurse Valerie Martin, on right, and home care provider Sonia Smith.

Hospice care in America has only been available for the past several decades, but for a family like that of Elene Gill, it was godsend. Long a sufferer of Parkinson's disease, Mrs. Gill spent her last months bedridden and incapacitated, but she was able to stay to the end in her home with her husband John—thanks to the palliative care provided by her nurse, Valerie Martin, of Washington Community Hospice. Valerie had help from Sonia Smith, who had given Mrs. Gill loving home care for several years.

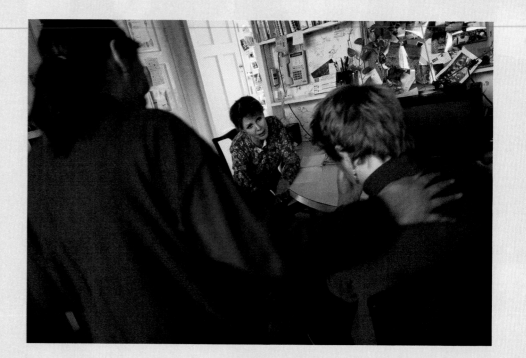

Saying her own good-byes to Mrs. Gill, Valerie gives her a kiss (below). "I always take time at the end to have my own personal moment with my patients." She also prepares the family (left), in this case Mrs. Gill's daughter, for the inevitable, telling them what to expect after their loved one passes.

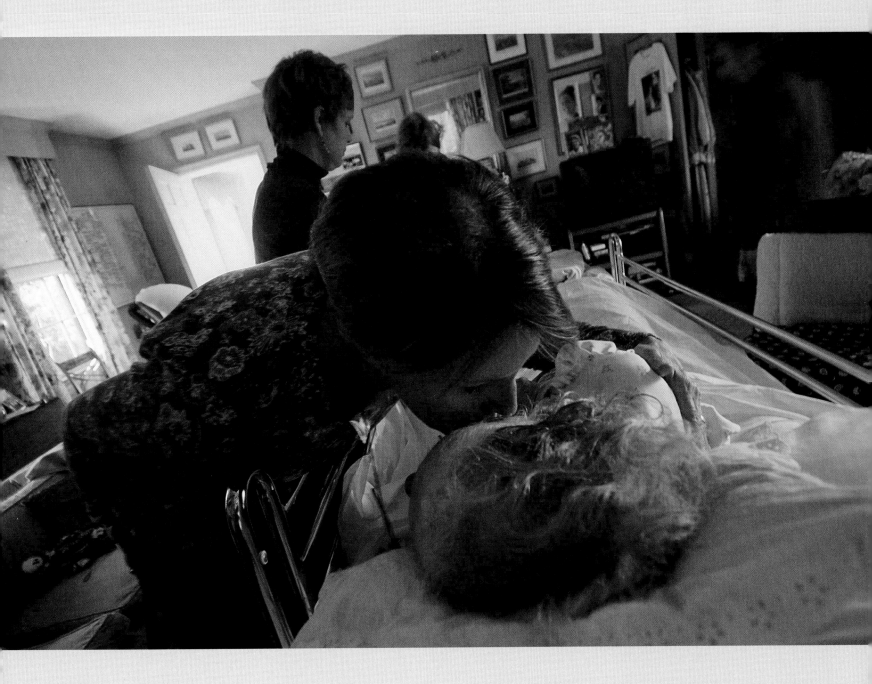

A KINDER PASSING

On her own, Sonia spends a quiet moment grieving for the patient and friend she took care of for years (below). Understanding Sonia's sense of loss, Valerie gives her an encouraging hug (bottom right). As the hospice nurse, Valerie must report the death (top right) to the patient's physician, and in D.C. to the medical examiner's office, before calling the funeral home.

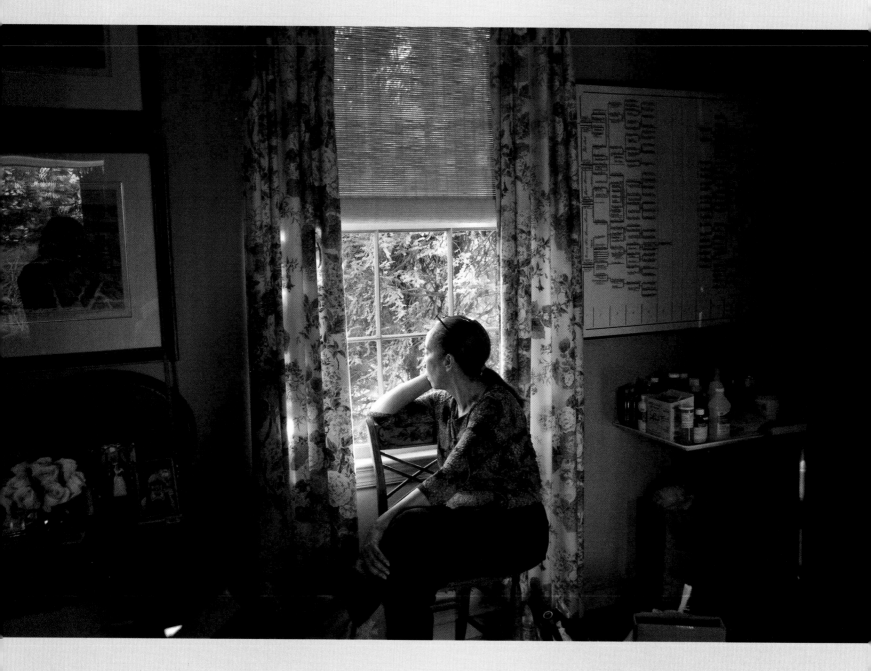

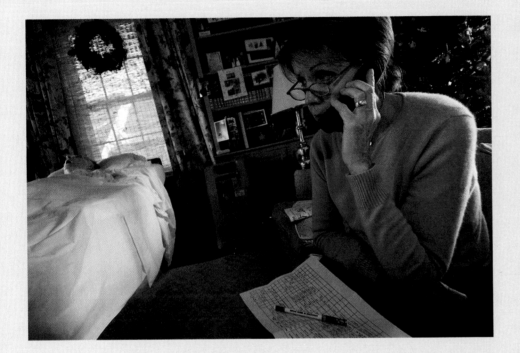

"Our culture has gotten away from teaching us to care for our own," Valerie Martin says. "But with hospice we show loved ones how to do that, and that knowledge and compassion for the dying gets passed down from generation to generation." Valerie has taken care of rich and poor, and she's seen firsthand, she says, that "death is truly the great equalizer. It's the responsibility of all of us—nurses, families, friends, and caregivers—to respect the dying for the full rich lives they've led and what they've given us. They deserve to die with the utmost love, care, and dignity."

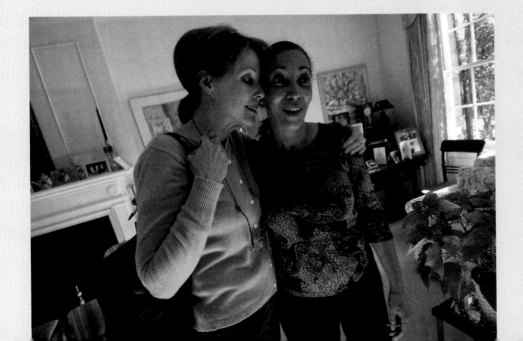

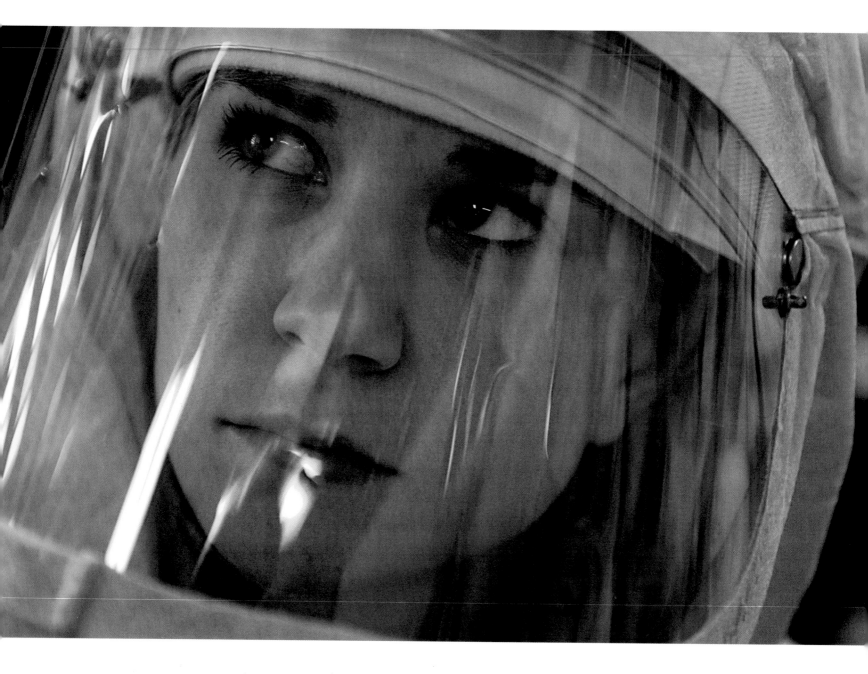

FIVE BRAVE NEW WORLD OF CARE

Necessity has always been the mother of invention among nurses. In rural Ethiopia, nurses lacking latex gloves wrap their hands with plastic bags to prevent passing infections from one patient to another. In Kingston, Jamaica, caregivers at the Missionaries of the Poor equip a plastic lawn chair with wheels so patients too sick to stand can receive showers. In a high-tech hospital in Houston, Texas, nurses put bright red booties on hospitalized patients who are at high risk of falling, so that everyone treating them will know to take extra care.

Today, nursing's spirit of determined ingenuity is taking on even bigger challenges, generating solutions to some of the most complex issues that health care has ever faced. Nurses are creating technology-based programs to enhance training, devising procedures to improve patient safety and the quality of care, launching media campaigns to encourage more young people to enter the profession, and designing state-of-the-art facilities that give nurses more time to care at the bedside.

Never before has the profession been so galvanized by a sense of mission and urgency. For good reason. Never before has nursing been so vital to the future of health care. In many cases, nursing *is* the future.

The face of the future, a nursing student is training for a world in which health care professionals will have to suit up to deal with biohazards posed by highly infectious organisms.

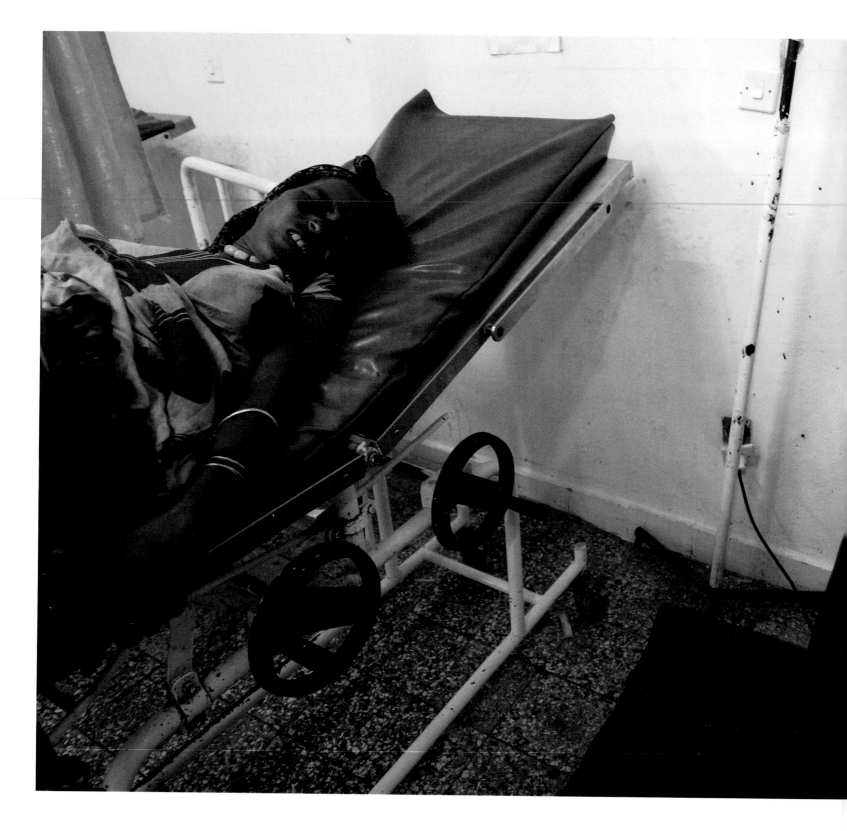

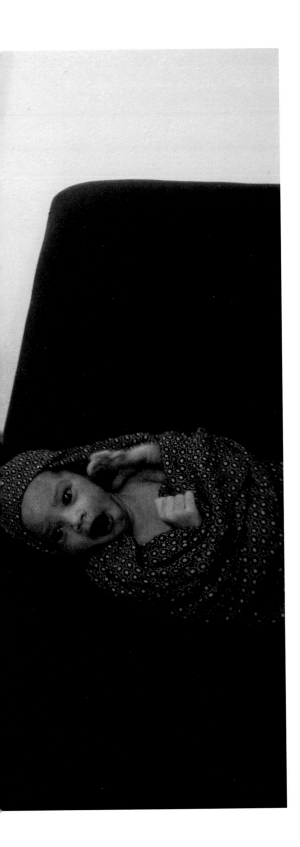

The worsening shortage of nurses in many parts of the world poses one of the most pressing challenges we face. And like any complex global problem, it will require a wide variety of solutions. One of them can be glimpsed in two small rooms at the Thika District Hospital, northeast of Nairobi, Ken-ya, where at almost any hour dedicated students work in front of glowing computer screens—part of an ambitious new software and Internet program designed to train more registered nurses. The computer center enables nurse assistants to earn degrees as registered nurses while continuing to work at the hospital, which desperately needs more trained nurses. Over a hundred such centers have been established throughout Kenya, and more than 2,000 prospective registered nurses are in training.

Other developing nations hard hit by an exodus of nurses have responded in their own unique ways. When a surge in migration left many critical-care units on the small island nation of Mauritius dangerously understaffed, nursing leaders knew the solution wouldn't be simple. "We had to act quickly to address the push factors—the reasons our nurses were leaving," said Francis Supparayen, a nursing policy expert in Mauritius. The first step was diagnosing the problem by means of a nationwide survey, which indicated that most nurses had emigrated to the U.K., drawn by higher pay and better opportunities. Because any solution bold enough to entice them to stay would require popular and governmental support, the

A long way from the high-tech world, this Ethiopian woman walked miles to ensure that her first baby would be delivered in a clinic—a rare occurrence for women in her region.

country's nursing association launched a media campaign to promote the importance of nursing. Capitalizing on the goodwill the campaign generated, they negotiated with the government to set up a comprehensive retention plan. Nurses are now allowed to work overtime and earn additional pay. They also receive an allowance to encourage them to stay in the country. The government agreed to increase recruitment at the country's two nursing schools from 70 to 300 nurses a year and is now developing an expanded nurse training program.

Not every battle has been won. In a previous wave of migration in the early 1980s, nurses migrated to Saudi Arabia and Qatar but eventually returned home, bringing valuable experience with them. Nursing leaders had hoped to encourage the latest departees to do the same by classifying them as "on leave without pay," which would allow them to return to work at their previous level. "The objective was to convert a brain drain into a brain gain through return migration," explained Supparayen. So far they haven't won that concession. Still, much has been accomplished. Nurses are now able to earn more money and pursue more opportunities. There is a greater sense among nurses that their work is genuinely valued and recognized. "Together, those changes have motivated them and encouraged many to stay," said Supparayen.

When Ghana, on the west coast of Africa, saw 300 of its nurses leave in 2002, leaders there pushed to increase salaries and offer nurses new career opportunities as well as educational options for their children. The government agreed to give nurses special access to loans for homes and for vehicles, which are vital to their work. A strong and vocal national nursing organization in Ghana helped push the reforms through.

These efforts, too, are paying off. In the first quarter of 2007, only two nurses left the country for work abroad.

In the face of a wave of outmigration, nursing leaders in the Caribbean decided to concentrate on recruiting and training more nurses. "We are a migratory people," explained Hermi Hewitt, who directs the School of Nursing at the Mona campus of the University of the West Indies, Kingston, Jamaica. "And there are important benefits to that for us. Migration in the Caribbean is typically circular, with people leaving to work abroad and then returning home, bringing valuable new experience." Hewitt herself has frequently gone abroad to study—at Harvard, the University of Iowa, and Tulane. By expanding educational opportunities, leaders decided, they could both fill positions left vacant by emigrating nurses and offer wider career opportunities to young people. A new Internet-based program for practicing registered nurses to obtain a baccalaureate degree in nursing was introduced at UWI, enabling these nurses to remain in their home countries while pursuing their education. A growing number of community colleges, both in urban and rural areas, have been encouraged to add nursing programs. "Many young people in the Caribbean dream of becoming nurses," said Hewitt. "We're working to make it more accessible for them to pursue that dream."

Ethiopia faces a far more daunting challenge. By the early 1990s, wrenching poverty and political instability had left much of the country's health infrastructure in shambles. The newly installed government began an ambitious program to build 500 primary care centers throughout the country. To help train nurses and other health care professionals to staff the centers, the Carter Center, with support from USAID,

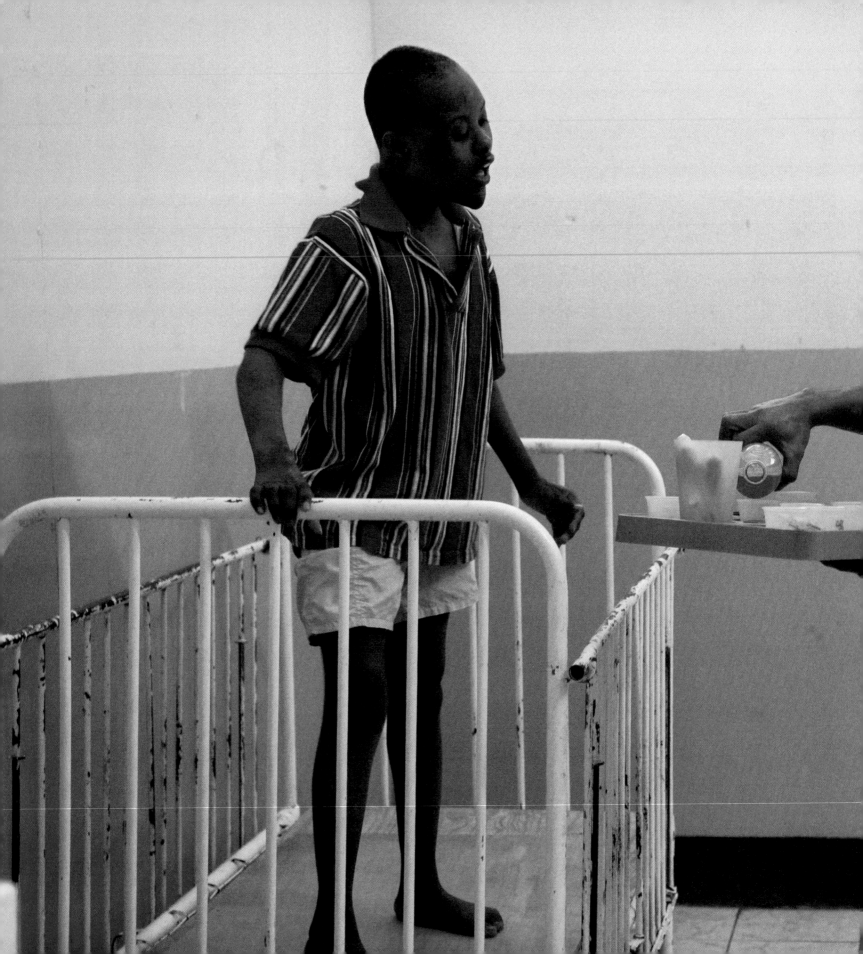

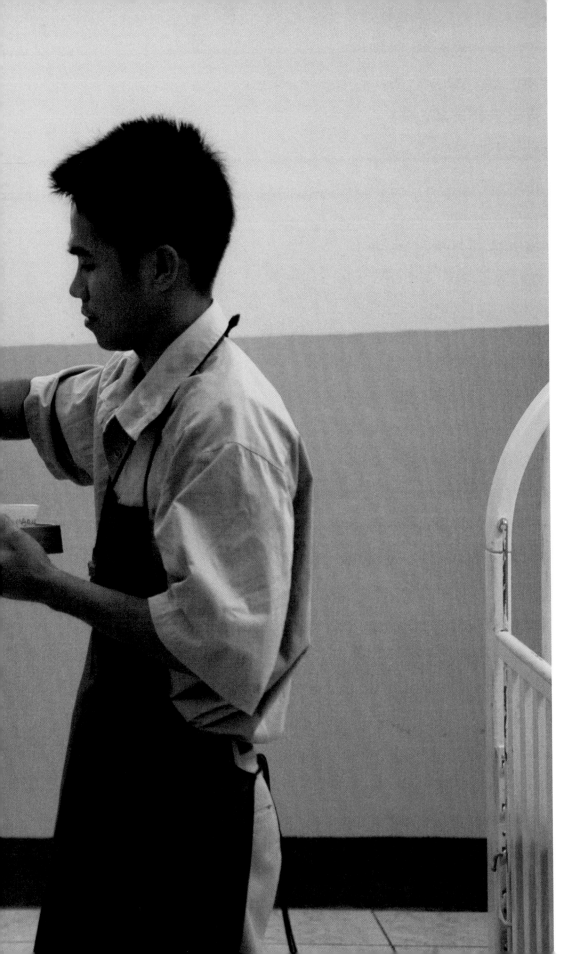

Challenged by severe mental and physical disabilities, a young Jamaican has found a simple but loving home with the Missionaries of the Poor, devoted to caring for those whom all others have abandoned.

began working with Ethiopia's Ministry of Health and Ministry of Education to expand and improve medical faculties at universities throughout the country. "Nurses are a major focus of the program because they play such a large role in health care in homes, villages, and communities in Ethiopia," explained Joyce Murray, who runs the Ethiopia Public Health Training Initiative for the Carter Center. "Nursing is all about caring, competence, and confidence, and that's what we're trying to build."

As a measure of its success, the Ethiopian government recently committed to building an additional 600 primary care centers, mostly in rural parts of the country. The goal is to graduate 5,000 health officers by 2011. Getting there will take hard work. "But one of the things we've learned," said Murray, "is that if you build a relationship of trust and respect with people, even in a place that's very different culturally and economically, you can accomplish almost anything."

SMALL COUNTRIES LIKE MAURITIUS AND GHANA CAN'T SOLVE THE PROBLEM OF migration alone, of course. The world's richest nations must also do their part. Here, the U.K. serves as a model. In the late 1990s, concerned about the consequences of migration, Britain's Department of Health published guidelines for the ethical international recruitment of nurses. One key provision, intended to prevent the plundering of poor countries' health workforces, stipulates that health professionals should be recruited actively by the National Health Service and the employment agencies that supply it only when there is an agreement with the sending country. Meanwhile, the U.K. began its own crash program to train more nurses and encourage those who were not practicing to return to the profession. "Letters went out to

The inequities and imbalances caused by global migration will never be fully resolved until the U.S. does a better job recruiting, training, and retaining its own home-grown nurses.

all nurses in England who were not working," explained Anna Maslin, an international nursing expert who has played a key role in shaping the U.K.'s international nursing workforce policies. "We offered free back-to-work courses to help nurses update their education and skills. At the same time, we made a significant effort to improve the working lives and career ladder of nurses." A government intiative called Modernizing Nursing Careers has gone a long way in opening up new opportunities for advanced-practice nursing and reshaping health care delivery to make the best use of nursing.

It's working. Six years ago, the U.K. imported more nurses than it trained. Today, the country is training enough nurses to be nearly self-sufficient. The WHO is currently creating a Code of Practice that would establish a general framework for ethical recruitment that could be used by countries around the world, both those that export and those that import nurses. "The goal is for sending countries and receiving countries to sit down at the table together and work out agreements that give nurses the freedom to work abroad while ensuring an adequate nursing workforce in the sending countries," said Jean Yan, PhD, Chief Scientist for Nursing and Midwifery at the WHO.

For now, the world's leading importer of nurses, the U.S., remains a powerful magnet—so powerful, in fact, that some experts insist that the inequities and imbalances caused by global migration will never be fully resolved until the U.S. does a better job recruiting, training, and retaining its own homegrown nurses. In 2002, to help jump-start that process, the global health care products company Johnson & Johnson joined forces with leading nursing associations to begin an unprecedented effort, called the Campaign for Nursing's Future. Its mission: to increase public

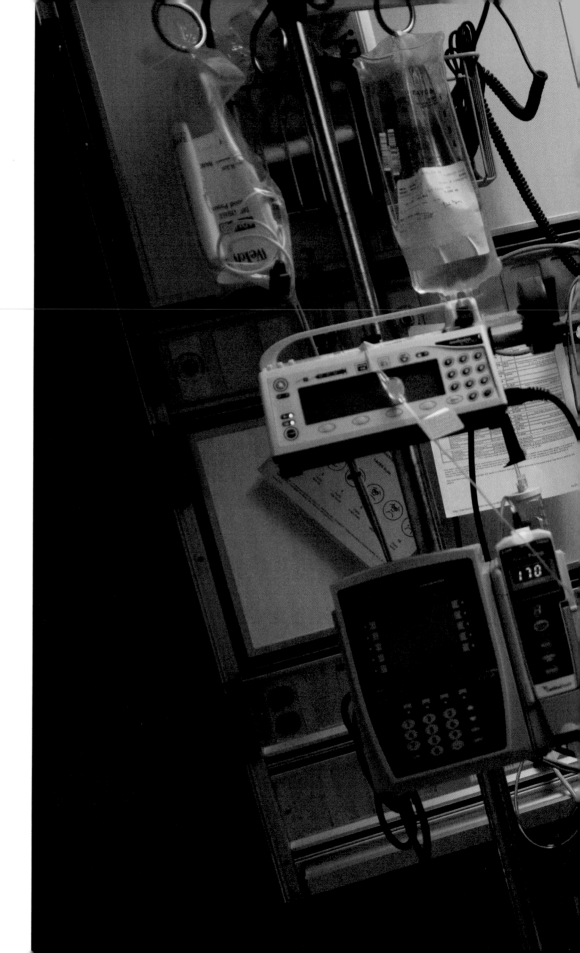

Machines deliver chemotherapy to a young cancer patient at a hospital run by Children's Health Care of Atlanta. In the U.S. and other wealthy nations, health care relies more and more on technology, but well-trained nurses are needed to manage the technology and provide the human face of health care.

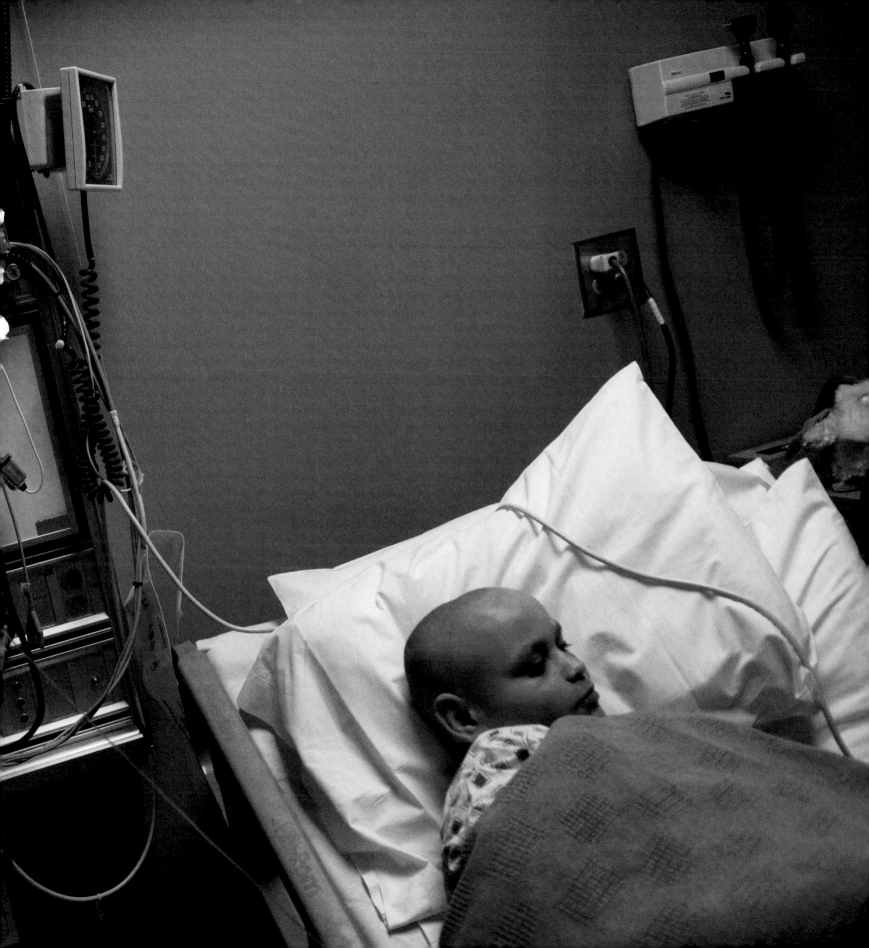

awareness of the importance of nurses and to attract more young people to the profession. One ad produced by the campaign shows nurses caring for a premature infant, a patient in an emergency room, and an elderly patient in a wheelchair. "This life was protected . . . this life was saved . . . and this life was made easier," the narrator says, "because of this life: nursing." In addition to television, radio, and print ads, the campaign includes an extensive website called discovernursing.com, which offers prospective nursing students information, including the world's largest database on nursing scholarships.

Nursing leaders credit the Campaign for Nursing's Future with enhancing the image of nursing and fostering a new understanding of its crucial role, encouraging others to step forward. In 2005, the U.S. Secretary of Education designated nursing as an "area of national need," making funds available to promote doctoral programs for nurses. In 2006, the American Association of Colleges of Nursing and the California Endowment announced a new scholarship program to attract more minority students to become nurse educators. A proposed "Troops to Nurse Teachers" program would offer incentives to retiring military nurses to join teaching faculties.

As essential as these initiatives are, they represent only part of the solution. More must be done to keep skilled nurses on the job. That means addressing the issues that have led many nurses to leave the profession early, from low pay and lack of respect to burnout caused by stressful and sometimes unsafe working conditions—a tall order by any measure. But here, too, a variety of innovations, many of them generated by nurses themselves, have fostered fresh optimism and growing excitement.

More must be done to keep skilled nurses on the job. That means addressing the issues that have led many nurses to leave the profession early, from low pay and lack of respect to burnout.

"MARY, WHAT'S YOUR COLOR, HONEY?" A SUPERVISOR ON THE MEDICAL-surgery unit of Seton Hall Medical Center in New Jersey asks.

"Green," one of the nurses responds. For the moment, at least.

Every few hours, the nursing team checks in to compare colors. Green means a nurse is doing fine. Yellow indicates she's really hustling and could use a little help if anyone's free. Red means she's overwhelmed and needs help ASAP

Color codes are just one of several innovations that have resulted from a groundbreaking program called Transforming Care at the Bedside, launched by the Robert Wood Johnson Foundation in 2003. "Why do nurses leave nursing?" asked Susan Hassmiller, who leads the program. "It's almost never the salary. It's poor working conditions. That's what keeps nurses from doing what they love to do and what they do best. Our task was to remove some of the barriers that prevent them from caring at the bedside."

The strategy is simple: enable nurses to get together to brainstorm new and better ways to deliver care—and give them the authority to implement them. As Hassmiller explained, "All ideas are welcome." Such brainstorming sessions led to the idea of a rapid response team, made up of a respiratory therapist and critical-care nurse who can respond at a moment's notice when other nurses recognize trouble. At the University of Pittsburgh Medical Center Shadyside, officials credit the rapid response team with saving 13 lives in one year. Another simple but effective change: putting brightly colored armbands and booties on patients at high risk of falling, to alert staff of the danger in case they wander off on their own. Several participating hospitals have also implemented "peace and quiet" time—a half hour every day when lights are dimmed

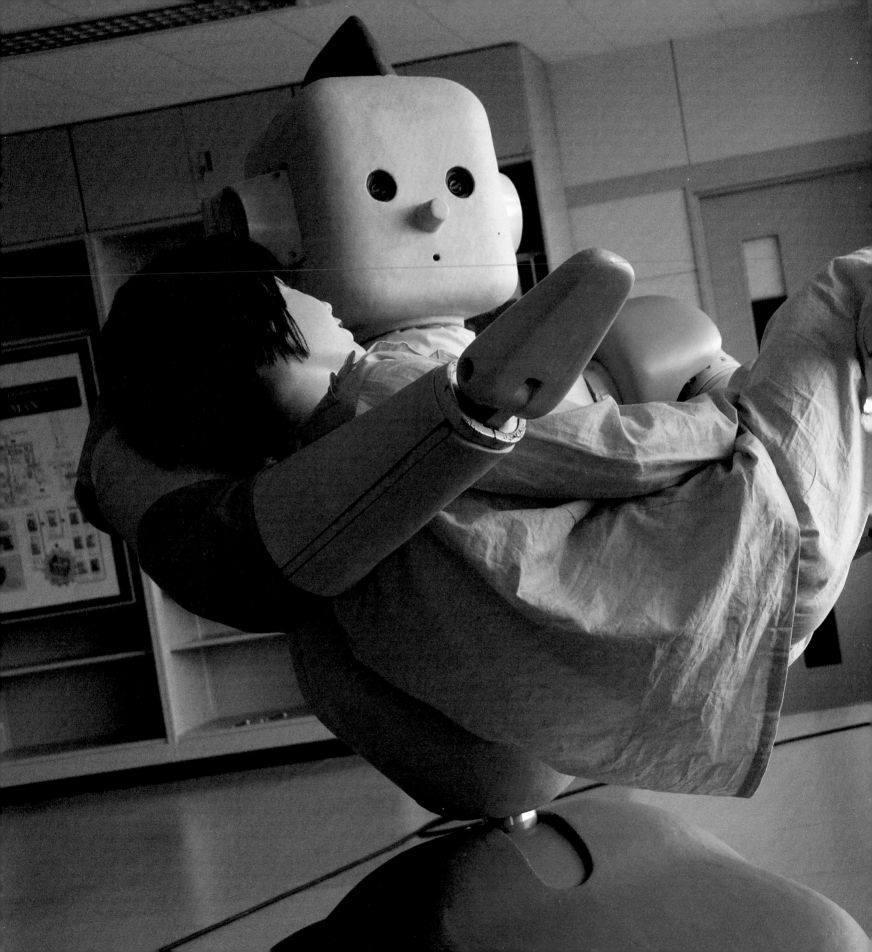

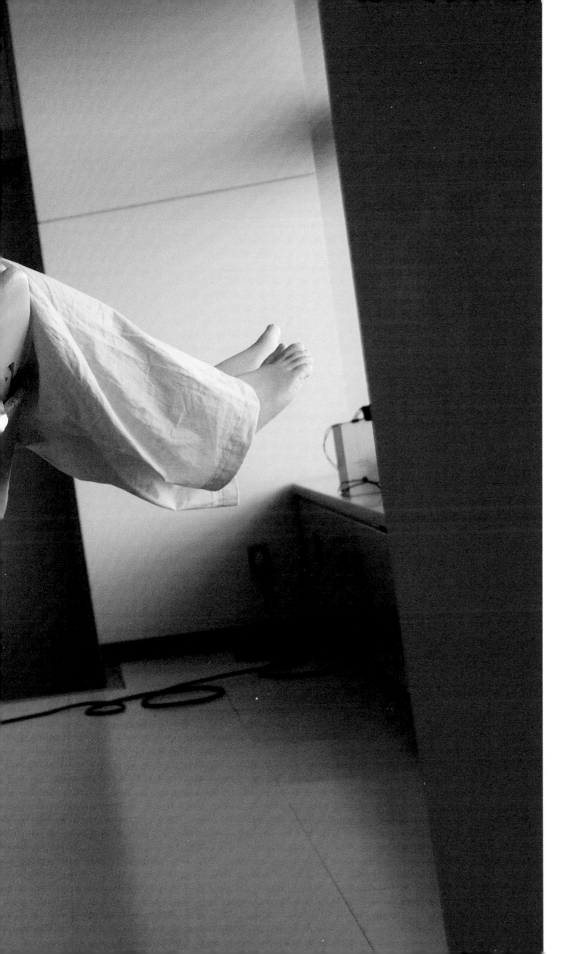

Not exactly a personal touch, but robots may be the future of health care. Japan in particular is engineering a variety of robotic caretakers, from lifters like this brawny model to human "washing machines." Robots could save wear and tear on nursing staffs and free up time for more critical decision making, but will patients adjust to non-human caregivers?

on the unit and soft music is played, providing a calming oasis for nurses and patients alike.

The success of Transforming Care at the Bedside can be measured in many ways. In most hospitals, nurses spend only 30 to 40 percent of their time at the bedside. Thanks to TCAB, nurses at participating hospitals spend more than 60 percent of their time directly caring for patients. That, in turn, has convinced many nurses who might have left the profession to stay on. Before instituting the program, the average voluntary turnover rate at participating hospitals was 15.5 percent. It's now under 5 percent. "I've been a nurse for years and years, and this is like nothing I've ever seen," said Seton Hall nurse Mary Johnston. "I actually chose the job that paid the least amount of money but gave me the most satisfaction."

Another innovative program is also convincing many nurses to remain in the profession. In 1983, the American Academy of Nursing's Task Force on Nursing Practice in Hospitals examined 163 hospitals in an effort to discover the features that attracted and retained top-flight nurses and promoted the best patient care. The task force identified 14 "forces of magnetism," including high levels of nurse autonomy, nurses serving as teachers, and an organizational structure and management style that promote innovative ways to improve care. In 1990, the American Nurses Association created the Magnet Recognition to award hospitals (and more recently nursing homes) that score well on all 14 variables. Almost 250 health care organizations now boast Magnet status. That coveted seal of approval, administrators have discovered, helps them attract and keep nurses on the job. At St. Joseph's Hospital Health Center in Syracuse, New York, vacancy rates fell from 19 percent in 2000, before Magnet status, to just 5 percent in 2007.

> "I actually chose
> the job that paid
> the least amount
> of money but
> gave me the most
> satisfaction."
>
> *Mary Johnston, Nurse*

Training more nurses and encouraging more to stay on the job will go a long way toward rebuilding the nation's nursing ranks. But most experts agree that even the most ambitious programs won't be able to meet soaring demand for nursing care over the coming decades. More must be done to enable nurses to expand their expertise and extend their reach.

Thanks to a growing sense of commitment and connection in the nursing community, that too is happening. For more than a century, the International Council of Nurses has given the profession strength and resolve. Its leadership continues to foster nursing's development and to expand the profession into new areas of concern, such as the well-being of female children around the world. In recent years the ICN has been joined by a growing range of new alliances. For example, under the auspices of the Lillian Carter Center for International Nursing, Government Chief Nursing Officers from around the globe convene to a biennial institute focused solely on their leadership development. Regional nursing alliances have also emerged as potent voices in addressing specific issues in places like the Caribbean, Central and South America, and Africa. Public-private partnerships are also building community and cooperation. Through its Global Health Fellows Program, for example, the pharmaceutical giant Pfizer matches experts on its own staff with organizations in the developing world. Many of its efforts focus on building a stronger and better-trained health care workforce.

As the Internet makes possible vast global communities on a scale never possible before, thousands of nursing-related websites, weblogs, and online communities have sprung up. In 2006, the WHO launched the Global Alliance for Nursing and Midwifery Communities of Practice—an

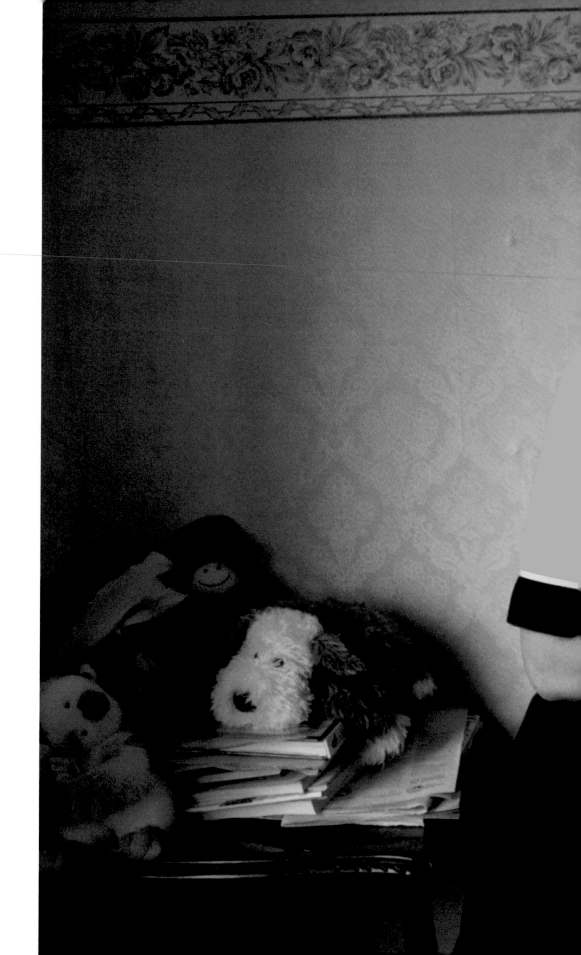

Caught in the web of her own
frightening deterioration, an
elderly Scottish woman relies on
the guidance and assurance of
her community health nurse,
who regularly checks on her in
her home. Increasingly, nurses
are the primary health care
providers for patients with little
or no access to physicians.

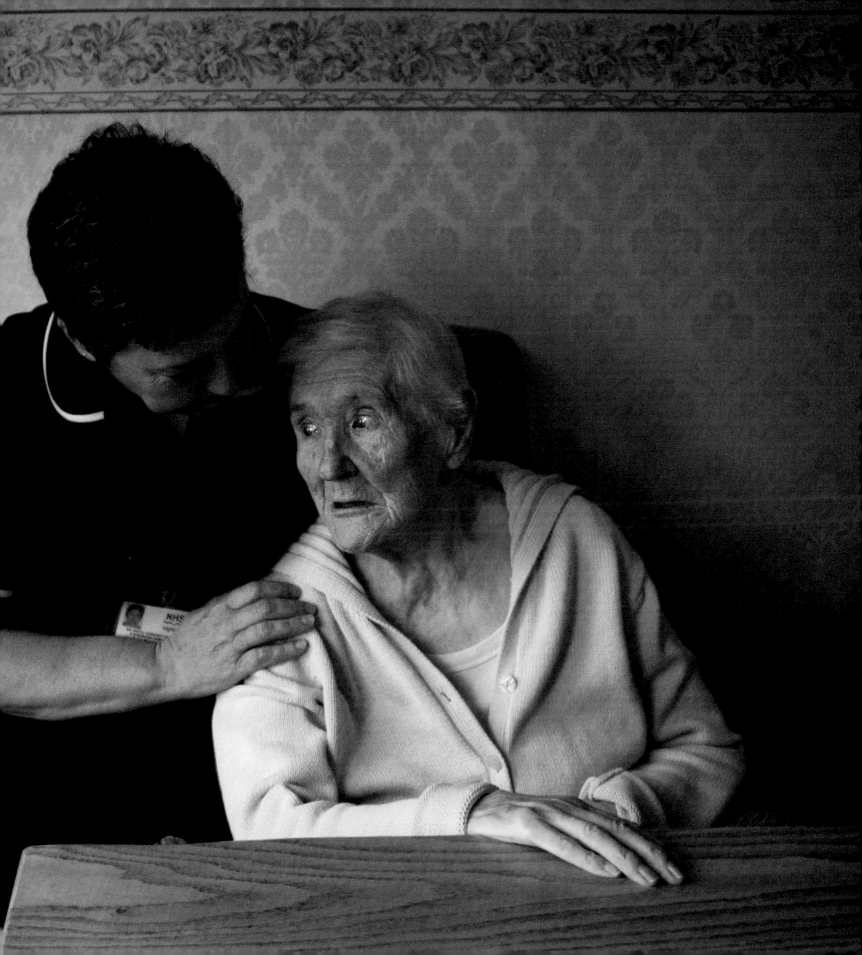

international forum for the exchange of ideas and experiences. The Alliance now has 1,300 members from 121 countries. "I recently heard from a nursing leader in a developing country who walked an hour to reach an Internet café so that she could participate in an online workshop," said the WHO's Jean Yan. "In another case, a nurse midwife in a rural area asked for assistance in developing standards of practice, and within 24 hours she had received six responses from around the world."

Other sites, large and small, are dedicated to everything from giving voice to nursing-related social activism to influencing the image of nursing in media. Nurses around the world are also tapping the power of telemedicine, extending their expertise across borders to serve people in remote and underserved areas via webcams and video technologies. In some cases, they're even participating in the planning and design of new health care facilities. In 2005, the new Saint Joseph's Community Hospital in West Bend, Wisconsin, opened its doors—a state-of-the-art facility designed specifically around patient care. Many of its innovations were inspired by nurses. To prevent falls, for example, bathrooms are placed as close to patients' beds as possible, with handrails along the route. Small alcoves placed adjacent to each room allow nurses to write up charts while keeping an eye on patients without disturbing them. By storing frequently used supplies in the alcoves, nurses cut down on "hunting and gathering" time, freeing up more time to spend in direct patient care. Nurses inspired the inclusion of family areas with fold-out beds, Internet access, and family storage closets in medical-surgery units and intensive care units—a feature showing up in more and more new hospitals.

Retirement communities and assisted living centers are also being

Technology has its limits, after all. Nursing still depends on human touch, a vigilant eye, a reassuring word, a receptive ear.

designed to make the most efficient use of nursing care. The Green House program, for example, creates homes for six to ten elderly people to live together, receiving support for daily activities and clinical care as needed but still retaining as much of their independence as possible. Communal kitchens and dining areas encourage a vibrant social life. In many hospitals and care facilities, sophisticated monitors linked to alarms enable nurses to respond within seconds when patients require critical care.

Even smarter technologies will transform nursing in the future. Infrared motion detectors can alert the nursing staff when a patient gets up and moves around at night, for example. A warning signal sounds if someone goes into the bathroom and doesn't return after a set period of time. Japanese technologists have even developed a person-size nurse robot that can lift and carry patients and deliver meals. The robot, which has soft hands and fingers that respond to touch, offers a promising solution to a problem many care facilities face: Back injuries, often sustained by lifting and moving patients, are a leading cause of disability among nurses and certified nurse assistants.

HELPFUL THOUGH THEY MAY BE, HOWEVER, ROBOTIC NURSES WON'T REPLACE their flesh-and-blood counterparts. It's not surprising, in fact, that the robots haven't proved as popular among elderly residents in Japan as their designers had hoped. Technology has its limits, after all. Nursing still depends on human touch, a vigilant eye, a reassuring word, a receptive ear. At Kolob Care & Rehabilitation Center in Saint George, Utah, resident Emery "Pete" Peterson, who has advanced diabetes, depends on the nursing staff to control his blood sugar levels and administer his medications,

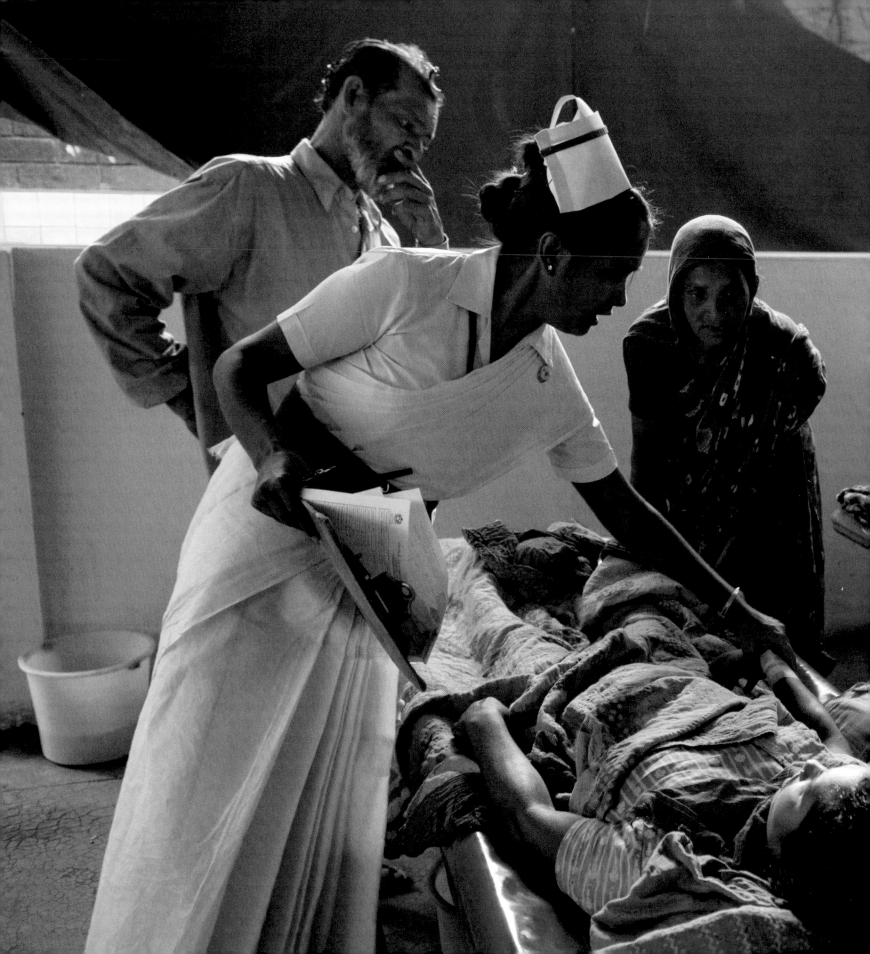

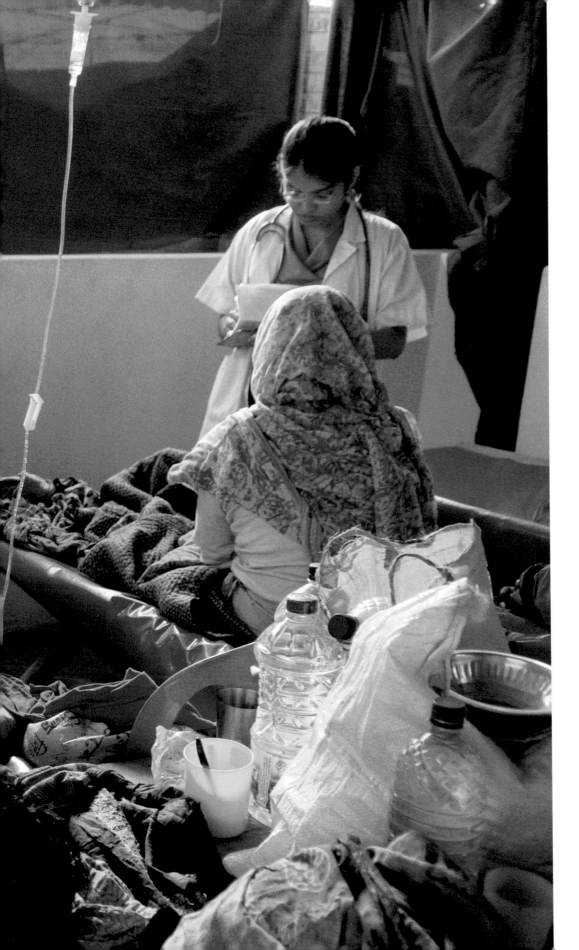

Weather disasters and even the normal change of seasons can bring death in undeveloped countries, particularly from diarrheal diseases. At the International Centre for Diarrhoeal Diseases Research, Bangladesh, nurses contend with cholera, usually affecting adults in the summer months; winter typically brings an outbreak of rotavirus infections in children. Often simple rehydration therapy is the only treatment required to save lives.

to get him up in the morning and into bed at night. His well-being relies just as much on the friendly banter and the occasional hugs the nurses give him when they make their rounds. As his wife, Mary, said, "You can just see his face light up when they come into the room."

Even as the profession of nursing looks toward the future, it is also returning to its roots, planted deep in the fertile soil of one-on-one patient care. Paul Martin, Chief Nursing Officer in Scotland, has helped pioneer a bold new model for nursing in the country, one that puts nurses front and center in efforts to improve health care. "One of the challenges we face in Scotland is our geography, a large landmass with many remote places," Martin explained. At the heart of the new program is the community health nurse, trained not as a specialist but as a generalist, someone who knows the community, someone who is equally at home treating a child with a fever or instructing older family members in how to care for a diabetic wound. Someone, in short, Florence Nightingale would have recognized immediately.

"Nurses make up about 70 percent of our health workforce, so they are an incredibly important resource," said Martin. "What we're doing is extending their contribution to reach more people by making community nurses the point of contact for health care. The goal is to provide care close to people's homes, even in their homes, and in places that may have had almost no access to healthcare before."

The family nurse program has gained traction not only in Scotland but in diverse communities around the world, from Finland and Iceland to Latvia and Estonia. Small wonder. Not long ago, experts in the School of Nursing, Midwifery & Community Health at Glasgow Caledonian University evaluated the latest pilot program in Scotland. Although their

Even as the profession of nursing looks toward the future, it is also returning to its roots, planted deep in the fertile soil of one-on-one patient care.

report is filled with impressive facts and figures, the most compelling testimony comes from the people served. Describing the community health nurse who now regularly comes by to visit, one respondent said, "She's always asking 'if you need any help any time, any time just give me a wee call, you know . . . just phone me any time.'" Another captured the way community nurses improve health care simply by dropping in and listening. "I think it's just things in general we could ask . . . . Sometimes my ma and da was in and they would ask her things. My dad had problems with his eyes and he asked her and she gi'ed him advice."

Similar programs have taken root in many parts of the world, offering nursing-based solutions to problems that once seemed intractable. In Lusaka, Zambia, for example, people with HIV/AIDS have found refuge in a remarkable place called Bwafwano. The name means "to help each other" in the local language. Working as a nurse, Beatrice Chola could no longer bear to watch people desperately ill with the disease being carried to a nearby clinic in wheelbarrows or on people's backs. Her heart had broken too many times listening to their stories of being stigmatized and sometimes abandoned because of their disease. Chola recruited and trained 50 women to work with her so they could visit patients in their homes. Eventually, she created the community of Bwafwano, where patients can live and receive care. By her example she has countered the widespread fear and discrimination that once surrounded the disease. "I made it very clear that AIDS is everyone's burden," she said. "I saw that, unless I involved the family, they would neglect the patient." Over the past decade, Bwafwano has grown into a vital community of care, with 280 nurses and caregivers looking after 1,300 people.

Programs like these, with their focus on community health and primary care delivered by nurses, represent a return to the enduring traditions of the profession. Yet in the context of today's high-tech medicine, they also offer a radical new way of thinking about health and well-being. Modern medicine has focused on treating people after they become sick, often in hospitals and at enormous expense. That model simply doesn't work in much of the world. And even where it currently holds sway, aging populations, the increasing burden of chronic disease, limited health dollars, and shortages of health care professionals make it increasingly difficult to sustain. Community nursing focuses instead on keeping people well and, when they become sick, enabling them to stay at home as long as possible, with their families, in their communities.

Of course nurses have long understood the importance of community and the simple fact that healthy communities are places where people can be healthy. For centuries they have been champions of self-care and preventive health. "Oh teach health, teach health, teach health," Florence Nightingale wrote in a private note in 1894, "to rich and poor, to the educated, and, if there be any uneducated, oh teach it all the more . . . ."

The future of nursing lies in the hands of the dedicated nurses who are empowering communities to improve their health and well-being. But just as important, it depends on the enlightened policies of governments and the active support of corporations and nonprofit health care groups. Indeed, everyone who might someday depend on the care and compassion of a nurse—every one of us, in other words—has a personal stake in a healthy future for nursing. Especially as health care takes center stage as a social cause and a political rallying cry, it's up to all of

Nursing is both
an art and a
science, a health
profession and
a calling, a set
of skills and a
sacred mission.

us to make sure that nursing receives due recognition, along with the resources it needs to remain vital and strong. "We simply must do more to give nurses the resources and the authority they need to lead, to shape policy and to make decisions," says the WHO's Jean Yan. "We must promote and nourish this profession if we are to address the inequities in access to health care and improve care for everyone."

AS THE PROFESSION LOOKS TO THE FUTURE, THE FUNDAMENTAL VALUES THAT have long guided nursing will serve as its compass. Nursing is both an art and a science, a health profession and a calling, a set of skills and a sacred mission. Nurses work with their hearts, hands, and minds. They are healers and counselors, teachers and consolers, tending not just the body but the spirit. Nurses must have knowledge and a high level of training, but those alone aren't enough. To be good at what they do, nurses must care, in the broadest sense of that word. Nurses care about individuals and families and communities, about babies not yet born and those in the last hours of life, about social justice and the right of everyone to a fair chance at a healthy life. They offer hope to the downhearted and encouragement to the dispirited. Through their vigilance and skill, they save lives. But even when there is no hope for a cure, when all they can do is offer compassion and consolation, they care.

"The things that nurses do really are miraculous," says Susan Grant of Emory University Hospital. "If nursing is to have a future, we must insist on giving value to the meaning of care. We must remember always that it is a sacred mission, caring for people at their most vulnerable. It takes someone very, very special to be a nurse."

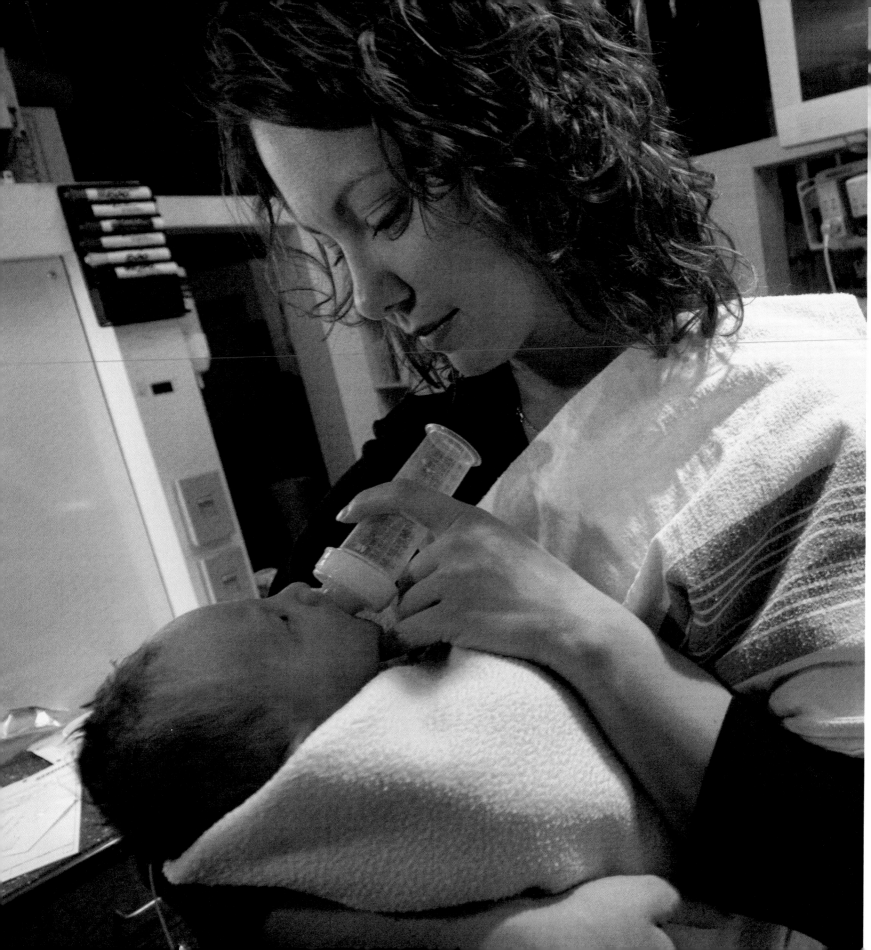

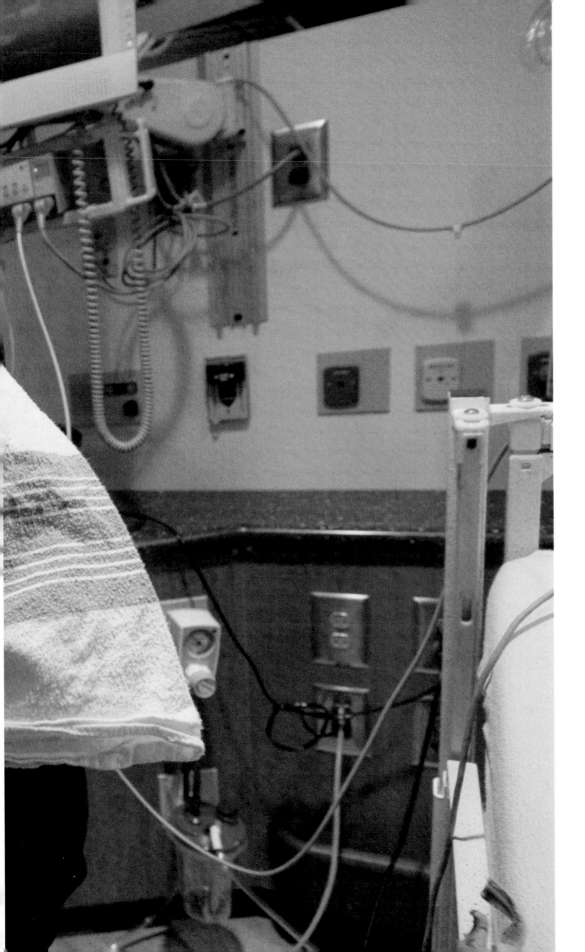

The promise of a new life triggers
the same elemental response across
borders, continents, and cultures.
But ensuring that babies grow to be
healthy, productive members of the
human race requires nurses—ever
there with skill and compassion,
care and commitment.

SOURCES

Chapter One

M. Patricia Donahue, *Nursing: The Finest Art, An Illustrated History,* C.V. Mosby Company, 1985

Dorothea Lynde Dix, *On Behalf of the Insane Poor*, University Press of the Pacific, 2001

David Gollaher, *Voice for the Mad: The Life of Dorothea Dix*, The Free Press, 1995

Massachusetts Foundation for the Humanities, State House Women's Leadership Project, "Dorothea Dix," 2001

Walt Whitman, "The Wound-Dresser," *Leaves of Grass*, 1867

Barbara Montgomery Dossey et al, *Florence Nightingale Today: Healing, Leadership, Global Action*, American Nurses Association, 2005

Florence Nightingale, *Notes on nursing: what it is, what it is not*, University of Michigan Library, 2005

Mary Seacole, *Wonderful Adventures of Mrs. Seacole in Many Lands*, Penguin Classics, 2005

Jane Robinson, *Mary Seacole: The Black Woman Who Invented Modern Nursing*, Carroll & Graf, 2004

"Mary Seacole," Wikipedia, www.enwikipedia.org

Salman Rushdie, *The Satanic Verses*, Viking, 1989

Lillian D. Wald, *The House on Henry Street*, Transaction Publishers, 1991

Henry Street Settlement, www.henrystreet.org

"Returning to Our Origins," Research Highlights, University of Virginia School of Nursing, www.nursing.virginia.edu/highlights

Mary Breckenridge, *Wide Neighborhoods: A Story of the Frontier Nursing Service*, Harper and Brothers, 1952

Melissa Gaskill, "Nancy Olivera, on nursing in Cuba," Nurseweek, December 4, 2001

Randy Shilts, "*And the Band Played On: Politics, People and the AIDS Epidemic*," St. Martin's Press, 1987

Lawrence K. Altman, "African Grandmothers Rally for AIDS Orphans," *New York Times*, August 13, 2006

Chapter Two

Barbara Montgomery Dossey et al, *Florence Nightingale Today: Healing, Leadership, Global Action*, American Nurses Association, 2005

Julie Fairman and Joan Lynaugh, *Critical Care Nursing: A History*, University of Pennsylvania Press, 1998

Claire Dennison, "Maintaining the Quality of Nursing Service in the Emergency Room," *American Journal of Nursing*, July 1942

"History of Nurse Anesthesia Practice," American Association of Nurse Anesthetists, www.aana.org

Phuong Ly, "A Labor Without End, *Washington Post*, May 27, 2007

Pol De Vos, "The functioning of the Cuban home hospitalization programme: a descriptive analysis," *BMC Health Services Research*, BioMed Central, May 2007

Lewis Thomas, *The Youngest Science: Notes of a Biology Watcher*, The Viking Press, 1983

Chapter Three

M. Patricia Donahue, *Nursing: The Finest Art, An Illustrated History,* C.V. Mosby Company, 1985

The Nightingale's Song: Nurses and Nursing in the Ars Medica Collection of the Philadelphia Museum of Art, Philadelphia Museum of Art, 2000

Barbara Montgomery Dossey et al, *Florence Nightingale Today: Healing,*

Leadership, Global Action, American Nurses Association, 2005. *Atlantic Monthly*, vol. 10, no. 60, October, 1862

Richard H. Carmona, "The Future of Nursing," Keynote Address at the National Student Nurses Association Conference, April 6, 2005, www.surgeongeneral.gov

Rooks et al, "Outcomes of care in birth centers: The National Birth Center Study," *New England Journal of Medicine*, December 28, 1989

Brooten et al, "A randomized trial of nurse specialist home care for women with high-risk pregnancies: outcomes and costs," *American Journal of Managed Care*, August, 2001

Bang et al, "Reduced incidence of neonatal morbidities: effect of home-based neonatal care in rural Gadchiroli, India, *Journal of Perinatology*, March, 2005

Bang et al, "Neonatal and infant mortality in the ten years (1993 to 2003) of the Gadchiroli field trial: effect of home-based neonatal care," Journal of Perinatology, March 2005

Judith Lupo Wald, et al, *Caring That Counts: The Evidence Base for the Effectiveness of Nursing and Midwifery Interventions*, Commonwealth Steering Committee for Nursing and Midwifery, May, 2003

Jagwe and Merriman, "Uganda: delivering analgesia in rural Africa: opioid availability and nurse prescribing," *Journal of Pain and Symptom Management,* May, 2007

"The Nurses Health Study," www.channing.harvard.edu/nhs/

Stampfer et al, "Primary prevention of coronary heart disease in women through diet and lifestyle," New England Journal of Medicine, July 6, 2000

Linda T. Kohn et al, editors, *To Err is Human: Building a Safer Health System,* Committee on Quality of Health Care in America, Institute of Medicine, National Academy Press, 2000

Ann Page, editor, *Keeping Patients Safe: Transforming the Work Environment of Nurses,* Committee on the Work Environment for Nurses and Patient Safety, Institute of Medicine, National Academy Press, 2004

Leape et al, "Systems analysis of adverse drug events: ADE Prevention Study Group," *Journal of the American Medical Association,* July 5, 1995

Aiken et al, "Hospital nurse staffing and patient mortality, nurse burnout and job dissatisfaction," *Journal of the American Medical Association,* October 23-30, 2002

Rafferty et al, "Outcomes of variation in hospital nurse staffing in English hospitals: cross-sectional analysis of survey data and discharge records," *International Journal of Nursing Studies,* February, 2007

Tourangeau et al, "Nurse Staffing and Work Environments: Relationships with Hospital-Level Outcomes," Canadian Health Services Research Foundation, March 2006

Tourangeau et al, "Impact of hospital nursing care on 30-day mortality for acute medical patients," *Journal of Advanced Nursing,* January, 2007

Needleman et al, "Nurse-staffing levels and the quality of care in hospitals," *New England Journal of Medicine,* May 30, 2002

Chapter Four

"Health Worker Shortage Limits Access to HIV/AIDS Treatment in South Africa," press release, Doctors Without Borders, May 24, 2007

"SOUTHERN AFRICA: Health staff haemorrhage limits AIDS treatment access," IRINnews.org, May 24, 2007

Laurie Garrett, "The Challenge of Global Health," Foreign Affairs, January/February 2007.

"Nurse Shortage Causes Chaos," *Australian Nursing Journal,* September 1, 2002.

Celia Dugger, "An Exodus of African Nurses Puts Infants and the Ill in Peril," *New York Times,* July 12, 2004

Mireille Kingma, *Nurses on the Move: Migration and the Global Health Care Economy,* ILR Press, Cornell University Press, 2006

Mireille Kingma, *Nurses on the Move: A Global Overview,* Health Research and Educational Trust, June 2007

Survey on the Future of Marin General Hospital, Marin Health Fund, July 12, 2005

Michelle Roberts, "Why I came to the UK to nurse," BBC News Online, 2004

Troy et al, "Nurses' experiences of recruitment and migration from developing countries: a phenomenological approach," *Human Resources for Health,* June 2, 2007

Working Together for Health, World Health Report 2006

Carlos Conde, "Philippine hospitals suffer as workers leave," *International Herald Tribune,* May 25, 2006

David L. Llorito, "Brain drain saps the Philippine economy," Asia Times Online, 2006

Stephen Bach, "International Mobility of Health Professionals: Brain Drain or Brain Exchange?" United Nations University, World Institute for Development Economics Research, 2006

Taking Stock: Health Worker Shortages and the Response to AIDS, WHO, 2006

What Works: Healing the healthcare staffing shortage, PricewaterhouseCoopers' Health Research Institute report, 2007

Anyangwe and Mtonga, "Inequities in the global health workforce: the greatest impediment to health in sub-saharan Africa," *International Journal of Environmental Research and Public Health,* June, 2007

Blendon et al, "Views of Practicing Physicians and the Public on Medical Errors," *New England Journal of Medicine,* Dec 12, 2002

Healthcare at the Crossroads: Strategies for Addressing the Evolving Nursing Crisis, Joint Commission on Accreditation of Healthcare Organizations, 2002

2003-2006 Enrollment and Graduations in Baccalaureate and Graduate Programs in Nursing, American Association of Colleges of Nursing

"What is the nursing shortage and why does it exist?" The Center for Nursing Advocacy, April 7, 2005

"Nursing Faculty Shortage Fact Sheet," American Association of Colleges of Nursing, www.aacn.nche.edu, October 4, 2006

Aiken, et al, "Nurses' reports on hospital care in five countries," *Health Affairs,* May/June 2001

2004 National Sample Survey of Registered Nurses, Health Resources and Services Administration, U.S. Department of Health and Human Services

Aiken, et al, "Hospital Nurse Staffing and Patient Mortality, Nurse Burnout, and Job Dissatisfaction," *Journal of the American Medical Association,* October 23/30, 2002

Ray Bingham, "Leaving Nursing," *Health Affairs,* January/February, 2002

"Nurses: love the job, but not the work environment," press release, International Council of Nurses, May 30, 2007

Chapter Five

"KENYA: Pioneering e-learning to boost nurse numbers," Medilinks, online at www.medilinks.org, October 24, 2007. Also available from IRIN PlusNews at www.plusnes.org

"Home Based Life Saving Skills: Where Home Birth Is Common," American College of Nurse Midwives, www.midwife.org

Campaign for Nursing's Future, www.discovernursing.com

"The Johnson & Johnson Campaign for Nursing's Future Crosses the Five-Year Mark," press release, Johnson & Johnson, May 9, 2007, www.jnj.com/news

"Troops to Nurse Teachers (TNT) Program," American Association of Colleges of Nursing, www.aacn.nche.edu

"Empowering Better Nursing Care: Transforming Care at the Bedside," online video, Robert Wood Johnson Foundation, www.rwjf.org

"Hospital Highlight: Seton Northwest Hospital," Robert Wood Johnson Foundation, www.rwjf.org

"Rapid Response Teams Becoming More Common in Hospitals," Robert Wood Johnson Foundation, www.rwjf.org

"Charting Nursing's Future," Robert Wood Johnson Foundation, April, 2007

"Transforming Care at the Bedside," Institute for Healthcare Improvement, www.ihi.org

"What is the Magnet Recognition Program?" American Nurses Credentialing Center, www.nursecredentialing.org, September 2007

"Forces of Magnetism," American Nurses Credentialing Center, www.nursecredentialing.org, October 2007

"Magnet status helps ORs attract and hold on to their nursing staff," *OR Manager,* June, 2007

Vian et al, "Public-private partnerships to build human capacity in low income countries: findings from the Pfizer program," *Human Resources for Health,* 2007, www.human-resources-health.com

Amy Eagle, "Better Safe," *Health Facilities Management,* December, 2007

Reiling, "Safe Design of Healthcare Facilities," *British Medical Journal,* 2006

Reiling, "Creating a Culture of Patient Safety through Innovative Hospital Design," *Advances in Patient Safety, vol 2.,* www.ahrq.gov

Pfizer Global Health Fellows Program, www.pfizer.com/responsibility/

"The Green House Concept," NCB Capital Impact, www.ncbcapitalimpact.org

"What is a Smart Home?", www.tiresias.org.

Graeme Wearden, "Robots could be nurses of the future," www.ZDNet.co.uk

RIKEN: Bio-mimetic Control Research Center, www. bmc.riken.jp

Barbara Parfitt et al, "An Evaluation of the Family Health Nurse Role, Phase 2," School of Nursing, Midwifery & Community Health, Glasgow Caledonian University, Final Research report, July 27, 2006

"Champions of care," *Where there's a will there's a way: Nursing and midwifery champions in HIV/AIDS care in Southern Africa*, Best Practices Collection, USAIDS, www.data.unaids.org

Barbara Montgomery Dossey et al, *Florence Nightingale Today: Healing, Leadership, Global Action,* American Nurses Association, 2005

INSTITUTIONS OF NOTE

The Carter Center
In partnership with Emory University, the Center works to advance human rights and alleviate unnecessary human suffering. Founded in 1982 by former President Jimmy Carter and former First Lady Rosalynn Carter and based in Atlanta, Georgia, USA, the center has worked in more than 70 countries.
Toll free in USA (800) 550-3560
international tel +1 404 420-5100
http://www.cartercenter.org

Commonwealth Health Ministers Steering Committee for Nursing and Midwifery
Part of the Commonwealth Secretariat, the London-based committee enhances the contribution of nurses and midwives to the health of the people of Commonwealth countries.
Tel + 44 (0) 20 7972 3959;
fax + 44 (0) 20 7972 4088
http://www.thecommonwealth.org

Global Network of WHO Collaborating Centres for Nursing and Midwifery Development
The network supports the contributions of nursing and midwifery in partnership with the WHO and its member states, centers, nongovernmental organizations, and others interested in promoting health.
Tel +41 22 791 2111; fax +41 22 791 3111
http://www.who.int

International Confederation of Midwives
The confederation, located in the Netherlands, supports and advises some 85 national midwifery associations in over 75 countries.
Tel +31 70 3060520; fax +31 70 3555651
http://www.internationalmidwives.org

International Council of Nurses
A federation of national nurses' associations in more than 128 countries, ICN works to ensure quality nursing care for all, enlightened health policies worldwide, and the advancement of nursing knowledge. It is based in Geneva, Switzerland.
Tel +41 22 908 01 00; fax +41 22 908 01 01; e-mail: cn@icn.ch;
http://www.icn.ch

International Federation of Red Cross and Red Crescent Societies
Based in Geneva, Switzerland, the world's largest humanitarian organization provides emergency aid and assistance throughout the globe.
Tel +41 22 730 42 22;
fax +41 22 733 03 95
http://www.ifrc.org

Johnson & Johnson's Campaign for Nursing's Future
Working in collaboration with nursing schools, health care organizations, and nursing organizations, the J & J program is designed to enhance the image of nursing, recruit new nurses and nursing faculty, and retain nurses currently in the profession.
http://www.Discovernursing.com or
http://www.Campaignfornursing.com

The Lillian Carter Center for International Nursing
Part of Emory University in Atlanta, Georgia, USA., the center is dedicated to the improvement of the health of vulnerable people worldwide through nursing education, research, practice, and policy.
Tel (404) 727-3130; international tel +1 404 72703130; fax (404) 727.9676
e-mail: lccin@nursing.emory.edu
http://www.nursing.emory.edu/lccin/

Sigma Theta Tau International
The honor society of nursing, STTI supports learning, knowledge, and professional development in nursing worldwide. Its offices are located in Indianapolis, Indiana, USA.
Toll free in USA (888) 634-7575;
international tel +1 317 634 8171
http://Nursingsociety.org

Social Transformation Programmes Division— Health Section Commonwealth Secretariat
Based in London, it assists member countries throughout the world in meeting goals that promote human development as the key to sustaining social and economic progress and achieving peace and democracy.
Tel +44 (0) 20 7747 6320;
fax +44 (0) 20 7747 6287
http://www.thecommonwealth.org

World Health Organization
An arm of the UN, the WHO supports initiatives to expand and improve nursing and midwifery around the world through the

office of the Chief Scientist for Nursing & Midwifery in Geneva, Switzerland, and through regional advisors for nursing and midwifery around the world.
Tel +41 22 791 2111; fax +41 22 791 3111
http://www.who.int

WHO Regional Advisors for Nursing and Midwifery
Africa Brazzaville, Congo;
Tel +242 839 100 or +47 241 39100,
fax +242 839 501 or +47 241 395018;
regafro@whoafr.org

WHO REGIONAL ADVISORS:
THE AMERICAS
Washington, D.C.; Tel +1 202 974 3000, fax +1 202 974 3663;
http://www.paho.org/

EASTERN MEDITERRANEAN
Cairo, Egypt; Tel +202 2276 50 00;
fax +202 2670 24 92 or 2670 24 94;
http://www.emro.who.int/

EUROPE
Copenhagen, Denmark;
Tel +45 39 171 717; fax +45 39 171 818;
http://www.euro.who.int/

SOUTH-EAST ASIA
New Delhi, India; Tel +91-11-2337 0804; fax +91-11-2337 9507;
http://www.searo.who.int/

WESTERN PACIFIC
Manila, Philippines;
Tel +63 2 528 8001;
http://www.wpro.who.int/

ACKNOWLEDGEMENTS

To the nurses of the world, this project is my way of honoring and thanking you for all that you do. To those nurses who have touched my life and exemplify all that is good about nursing, to those who believe in them and support their work, a special thanks. Among them, Lillian Carter, whose legacy continues to inspire and engage—and whose son President Jimmy Carter deeply understands the meaning of caring. To my mother, Marceline Salmon, RN, who paved a steep path for two subsequent generations of nurses, and to my dad, Everett Salmon, MD, whose respect and love for nurses was unwavering. To two wonderful nurses who have literally made a world of difference, Professor Anna Maslin and Dr. Jean Yan. And to my incredible, funny, patient, and inspiring family—my husband Jerry; my children, Jessica and Matthew; and my grandson, Parris. I love you all so much!

To my closest collaborators, Karen Kasmauski, Peter Jaret, and Bill Douthitt—you are giants. From the very beginning, your commitment and talent have inspired and sustained me. And to Dianne Winsett, my closest Emory partner, who has shown unwavering belief in this project, despite having to knit together all of those loose strings.

A very special thanks to the Johnson & Johnson Company for the critical support that has helped to make this project possible. Their Campaign for Nursing's Future has advanced the profession of nursing around the world. Andrea Higham, the campaign's leader and nursing's best friend, has been generous in her enthusiasm and wisdom throughout this process. I join millions of nurses in my gratitude to you and to Johnson & Johnson.

To our many, many friends and partners around the world who have made this project possible—and to our team, Karen Kostyal, Bob Gray, and Laura Reynolds; I am forever in your debt.

Special thanks also to the faculty and students of the Nell Hodgson Woodruff School of Nursing at Emory University, who gave so much to this project—and to Chris Kellner, Emory attorney and champion; Susan Eckert; Kathy Kite; Roman Damena; Teresa Fosque; Steve Hochman; Rick Luce; and so many other people who generously pitched in when most needed. To our student fact checker-researcher-remarkable person, Karen Thomisee; you are just great! And to Emory, where doing good actually matters—thank you.

Carla Hall, you'd make a great nurse midwife—thank you for believing and partnering. Thanks also to Kathy Bennison, Jeff Burnham, and all at Sigma Theta Tau who have pitched in.

OK, everyone. Thanks to you, we did it!

Marla Salmon

Being part of this amazing project has been a blessing and a privilege, and there are so many people to thank that it's difficult to know where to begin. First and foremost, I want to thank Bill Douthitt, my collaborator on this project, and my partner, confidant, husband, and best friend. I am a better person because of him. I also want to thank our two children, Will and Katie, who, as usual, had to put up with their mom being on the road somewhere.

I also want to express my gratitude to Marla Salmon, the Dean of Emory University's Nell Hodgson Woodruff School of Nursing, who asked me to help make this project a reality. Her assistant, Dianne Winsett, held the project together and was always there to address my questions, and Patty O'Connor got me where I needed to go in the shortest and safest way possible. Also from Emory, I want to thank all the members of the teaching staff and student body who put up with me and let me photograph them at work. Among these, I'd particularly like to acknowledge Maureen Kelly, Joyce Murray, Linda Spencer, Judith Wold, Martha Rogers, Suse Zughaier, and Pat Riley.

A project of this magnitude cannot be completed without the kind and generous support of people throughout the world. So many nurses, administrators, doctors, caregivers, families, and others involved in various health projects contributed to making my journey smooth and fruitful that I can only list a few by name. But to all the others who helped, and particularly those featured in the photographs in this book, I send my sincere thanks.

Among those whose help was invaluable are Jean Sacks, who made things happen in Dhaka, Bangladesh; Dr. David Sacks, former director of ICDDRB, and all the staff at ICDDRB, Dhaka, Bangladesh; Father Richard Ho Lung, founder of the Missionaries of the Poor; Dr. Dennis Carlson, who introduced me to Sister Yewaganesh, HAPCSO, Addis Ababa, Ethiopia—and thanks to HAPCSO founder Sister Tibebe; Ruth Lubic, founder of the Healthy Baby Birthing Center in Washington, D.C., Diana Jolles, director of the center, and all the nurse midwives and moms I worked with there; Staff at Washington Community Hospice and particularly Valerie Martin; Montgomery County Schools, Maryland, which allowed us to photograph the school nurse and family care program; Barbara Gibson and staff at Frontier Nursing Service, Wendover, Kentucky; Gloria Peña, Chief Nurse, and her staff at the Laredo, Texas, Public Health Service; Sister Angela, founder of the Family Health and Birthing Center in Weslaco, Texas, and her midwives, nurses, and moms; Nikkei National Geographic, Tokyo; Officials at the Nanto City Department of Health and Welfare, Japan, and Kunio Kadowaki who facilitated my trip to Japan; Jennie Chin Hansen and the staff from the various On Lok facilities in San Francisco; Cynthia Hernandez, Director of the Ellenton Health Clinic, Moultrie, Georgia, and José Palomare who opened the door for me to the migrant community in Moultrie; the Samaritans of Arizona and the people who work with them; Marilyn Elegado-Lorenzo, Manila, Philippines, who made nursing contacts for me throughout the country; Maria Daniella Lancini who introduced me to many communities in Venezuela; Dr. Jacinto Convit, Director of the Biomedical Institute, Caracas, Venezuela; Staff of Children's Health Care of Atlanta, Georgia; Rhonda Richtsmeier, Chief Nurse, and the other nurses I worked with in the Alaska public health system; Ruth Ota, Chief Nurse, and the other nurses I worked with in the Hawaii public health system; Staff at the following Hawaiian institutions: the Queen's Medical Center, Oahu; the North Hawaii Community Hospital on the Big Island; the Waianae Coast Comprehensive Health Care Center, Oahu; and Cynthia Rankin, Regional Director of Public Relations for Hilton Hawaii; Monique Petrofksy and others at CDC who have helped with ideas and contacts, and Mark Simmerman, CDC, Bangkok, Thailand; Staff at Ben San Leprosy Treatment Center, Vietnam, and Father John Toai and the pastoral care staff from the Roman Catholic Diocese of Ho Chi Minh City; Staff of the National Health Service in Scotland who helped move this project along, including Chief Nurse Paul Martin, Jane Walker, and Pat Tyrell; Khitam Barqaw who hosted me and facilitated my work in Amman, Jordan, and Dr. Hanan who helped me locate Palestinian nurses; Agnes Waudo, the former Chief Nurse of Kenya, and the current Chief Nurse, Chris Rakuom, and especially to Jael Waswa, who introduced me to the nursing outreach community in Nairobi.

Karen Kasmauski

I am grateful to a very long list of people who generously took time out of busy schedules and away from more important duties to talk to me about their work and the role of nursing around the world. If this book succeeds, it is because of their passion, commitment, and inspiration. I also owe a debt to the researchers, journalists, and writers whose published work I consulted in order to give this book its substance and scope.

A book like this is a collaboration, and I had the good fortune to be part of an exceptional team. I'm very grateful to Karen Thomisee, who checked the manuscript for accuracy and balance while finishing her degree in nursing, and to Karen Kostyal, both for her superb editing and for making this project a pleasure from beginning to end. I want to thank Bill Douthitt for pushing the project along with an unwavering sense of humor, Bob Gray for gracefully balancing words and pictures, and Dianne Winsett for assisting at the drop of a hat. Marla Salmon's wisdom and nurturing touch are reflected on every page.

Finally, thanks to Sue Licher, Susan Jaret McKinstry, Jack and Sally Jaret, and Michael Jaret and Jacqueline Smith for their encouragement. And a special thank you to Steven Peterson for listening patiently to a lot of half-formed ideas and putting up with too many working weekends.

Peter Jaret